The many Faces of M.E./CFS

Real, Raw, Short Stories by Actual Patients

Susan Parker Rosen & Donna Short RN

The many faces of M.E./CFS

Real, Raw, Short Stories by Actual Patients

By Susan Parker Rosen & Donna Short RN

ISBN: 9781712072608

Book design by Invisible Publications

Published by Invisible Publications

Copyright 2019 – Invisible Publications

This book is dedicated to Salesian Sisters (Sr Mary Rinaldi, Sr Liz Ryan and Sr Mary Zito) as their continuing prayers have led me to find acceptance and healing. Their lovely prayers led me towards my calling; books on Invisible Disorders such as ME/CFS and Fibro.

God Bless
https://www.salesiansisters.org/
Susan Parker-Rosen

Table of Contents

Introduction

"ME/CFS Awareness Means No More Sweeping Chronic Fatigue Syndrome Under the Rug." ~**Susan Parker Rosen**

Myalgic encephalomyelitis/chronic fatigue syndrome (ME/CFS) patients, those that struggle daily with a depilating disease will find others telling stories of similar symptoms within these pages. Our hope is that those that have someone else in their lives with this syndrome will also find that the struggle is very real. Actually, it's been noted in this publication, that the symptoms are so similar that it's highly unlikely the shared symptoms are not authentic. Think about it, two different people, living on other sides of the world would complain of the same constant exhaustion along with sore swollen glands, that never ceases nor improves. They also struggle with other symptoms that are very similar. That begins the unraveling of the disease's mask; that has been diagnosed in the United States dating back to as far as 1934.

Yet today, as of this writing, it still is not treatable by the medical community in this country. Unless someone has been cut off from the internet, most of the public is familiar with the many online groups that are almost commonplace for those of us with varied invisible Illnesses. Our ME/CFS 'go to' groups are where those of us that struggle can find others with the common-place symptoms that we face. With all the groups out there that are so easy to find, why would someone want to read this publication? Simple. Our series of books tie the two worlds together, the world of the person that struggles with ME/CFS and those who do not. Most online groups are closed off to the general public which is understandable for all those that want privacy. Invisible diseases carry a stigma, since people cannot actually "see' that we are ill, and therefore have a hard time empathizing with our horrid symptoms.

These books are designed to connect all types of people that struggle with those that do not struggle. We connect the dots by telling our personal struggles in raw short stories. Most of the stories you'll read are heartfelt, and you'll not only want to read through yourself, over and over, you will be gifting these books to your friends and relatives. You do not need to have this syndrome to feel the pain in our writers' voices. Nor to feel the exhaustion, as it probably took them a little longer than a healthy person to craft each one. But each and every book we publish contains honest stories and can be very inspiring to all of us, whether you struggle with an invisible disease or not.

A little about Invisible Publications. In 2018 we began putting our first fibromyalgia book together. We came together on Social Media to spread awareness one story at a time. I had an idea that what we see and read in our online groups should be available within a books page's in a transparent and honest way. The first book in the series, "The Many Faces of Fibro," was born. When we decided to craft our second book in the series the excitement began to spread. Now we can be heard, now our voices will not be ignored. Writers became excited as we started to swim in unchartered waters. We are all taking off our masks to cover our illness and allowing the world to witness us open and raw.

Our team never dreamed that our books would go this far but we knew that we wanted to spread awareness we must connect the insight found within our support groups to the printed and digital world. Since that time, we have mushroomed in size. We now have 4 books published to date (this being the 4th). A few books are in the pipeline for publishing very soon. Our plan is to have many more books published in our series. We hear from several real sufferers almost daily, asking for information on how they too can tell their story within our pages. Our writers have grown in numbers with many writings for our multiple books. Many have said that they enjoy, not only reading but also crafting pieces for our publications, as it has brought them healing in their journey with Invisible Illnesses.

Think of us as the "Chicken Soup for the Soul," for Invisible Illnesses. Giving each and every person the opportunity to have a voice to talk about their life and how their invisible illness/es has affected them. Not just a voice, but a published voice. This is offered at no cost to the writers! The entire team that put this book together works hard every day to spread awareness, that is our main objective.

So much happens behind the scenes that it's almost impossible to list the duties we perform to get these books to print. Once stories come in, we organize and edit each story. Edited stories become organized and then the process for formatting and publishing begins. Along the way we create support groups in Social Media for our writers, we hold contests and have so much fun! I would love to have you join us in one of our groups' (listed in the back page) to meet some of our writers, or some of those that work on our team to bring you these stories.

The team at Invisible Publications are all struggling from an invisible illness ourselves; supporting each other as we work. Most of us struggle with both fibromyalgia as well as ME/CFS. We have found that by writing about our lives, writing about not only our feelings, but of our disorders and diseases, that we begin to find healing. We also find that by publishing these books other people become aware of our specific challenges. It's a simple concept: one person telling the story has power, but what about 5 people, or 10 people or 25+ people telling the story of the symptoms, including sore and swollen glands in various places of the body as well as feeling your body shut down, yes this literally does happen if you try to exert yourself too much.

As you will begin to read through the individual stories you'll enjoy that we present them in the kindest, sweetest, honest light that will encourage even the healthiest of people to want to read our books, they want to learn about ME/CFS. Most importantly, we want the people in the life of the ME/CFS sufferer to read these stories, that's where the real magic of these books unfolds.

The vision for these books is that there is strength in numbers. That we want our writer's stories available in libraries, doctors' offices, on your husband's or wife's nightstand, a gift to a family member, who (excuse me) tried and just doesn't "get-it," That is how we can make a difference, it's one thought, one effort and one story at a time. No one will know about the personal lives with this illness and what it did to change them forever unless these short stories are written. We encourage our writers to talk from the heart when they write, the stories pour in and then voila the book is published!

For my personal story, I was ill with CFS for 26 long years until I stumbled upon relief. In fact, I very rarely need to take another supplement. Other natural medications have assisted in my struggle.

That testament is included within. Prior to this book going to publishing I had my first ME/CFS flare in a long time due to personal stress, that brought the pain and the horrid exhaustion flooding back into my current memory. Sometimes we forget about the pain, oh we remember it's painful, but we forget the exact pain. This flare was not mistaking it, the pain in the joints, the excruciating stabbing pain that I felt, also while I was so exhausted and having a hard time pushing through my day. My brain wasn't firing any pistons, in fact I felt brain dead!

More concerning my stories are included in these pages, as well as our co-author Donna Short RN's stories. As promised, many other writers' stories should help you the reader, to relate to many circumstances in your life or in the life of someone you know with this horrid syndrome. Even though there is validation, there is no medication that has been introduced by the medical field (that we know of at the writing of this book) that can neither cure nor combat the symptoms of ME/CFS.

Now let me get my venting over while I can, as many of us with invisible illnesses do too often. Let this sink in for a moment: There is no pharmaceutical medication to date, that the medical field has introduced to counteract the virus nor it's numerous symptoms. And yes, it appears to be a viral infection. Why is this so mysterious and where did ME/CFS start as the first known cases?

I went on a mission to find out some history about our somewhat unknown syndrome. As I mentioned in the beginning of the introduction ME also known as Myalgic Encephalomyelitis was first diagnosed in the United States in 1934. I found some excellent information in MePedia.com. In 1948 in Iceland more were diagnosed, many more in 1955 Royal Free Hospital in London, also the most infamous, the 1984 cases in Nevada (also clusters at the same time in NYC. As a side note, I contracted this in 1984 while I resided in Philadelphia and worked for a company with many NYC clients in and out.).

To worsen matters and muddy the waters Mia Farrow who was diagnosed with Polio has a blog and with more information on how ME/CFS and Post-Polio Syndrome can be tied together. I was aghast when I read this excerpt written by Mia:

WHAT ARE POST-POLIO SEQUELAE?

"Post-Polio Sequelae (PPS, Post-Polio Syndrome, The Late Effects of Poliomyelitis) are the unexpected and often disabling symptoms -- overwhelming fatigue, muscle weakness, muscle and joint pain, sleep disorders, heightened sensitivity to anesthesia, cold and pain, as well as difficulty swallowing and breathing -- that occur about 35 years after the poliovirus attack in 75% of paralytic and 40% of "non-paralytic" polio survivors. There are about 2 million North American polio survivors and 20 million polio survivors worldwide. The existence of PPS has been verified by articles in many medical journals, including The Journal of the American Medical Association, the American Journal of Physical

Medicine and Rehabilitation and The New England Journal of Medicine."

You can locate the remainder of Mia's article at the following website referenced:

www.cfstreatmentguide.com/blog/post-polio-syndrome-and-mecfs-common-ground

Wow, there are a few symptoms in there that many fibromyalgia patients describe often as well. Especially the difficulty swallowing. That one really hit home. The website also highlights that exercise is our enemy and can cause more harm. How many people in your life have suggested you get more exercise? Make sure you respond with a reference to our book, and that they need to read this particular copy. If a physician has suggested that you do more than is comfortable, they too should also read a copy of this publication. As it is documented in most references, regardless of what they call our illness, exercise can and will make our symptoms worsen. Our reasoning for these books can go deeper then spreading awareness we are also sending a message to the medical industry. We are growing in numbers and it's time to find answers. Real answers. The community of disease control is also being addressed; they need to help us break through, not only the stigma, but the mystery behind this syndrome.

When I contracted ME/CFS in 1984 I had no one to talk to about this illness, there wasn't social media, in fact there wasn't an internet that we know of today. I was confused as to what was happening to me medically and really had no answers. Luckily, my mother had been given a very brief magazine article about the new and mysterious

"Yuppie Illness" and how it was 'for life.' The article was very short and to the point, there was no doubt in my mind that I struggled with that same illness. That article was the only thing I had, the only thing to hold on to back in the 80's.

No one could possibly understand what I was going through. Isolation started to ensue. No one else that could even fathom what I was living with in terms of constant exhaustion and horrid swollen glands as well as fevers, night sweats and sore throats. I was always, always sick. Now, I didn't have any information at the time to substantiate the symptoms of M.E., but I always felt as if I was coming down with something or was definitely ill. Never feeling quite right, I still had to work. Later possibly fibromyalgia due to trauma from a major car accident. I lived with both, worked full-time for quite some time.

For those that do suffer with this syndrome, the internet, and frankly Facebook has become, at least for most, our sole connection to the outside world and a way to meet others that also fight the fight with this exhausting and life changing syndrome. As many problems as Facebook may create for some situations, it also solves and brings so much good into our lives. So many of us that are ill, housebound or even unable to connect with others that complain of the same symptoms and that have the same frustrations.

In my circumstance, I didn't know anyone else in the mid-eighties that was diagnosed with this syndrome. Can you imagine the stigma I felt back then as you think of the stigma now that it's 35 years later? And honestly, as I'm writing this, I'm not sure if the stigma changed. To this day, I probably only have known one person with ME/CFS.

Yet, I have many internet friends that struggle, they are now the people I know personally. You bet they are. They have become my best friends in this journey called life. I hope that I can offer them the same love and comradery that they have offered me. This is also what I wish for everyone that struggles and hasn't found their tribe. People that know each and every day that you are in pain and they care.

Trying to be normal while living with a stigma, a life changing syndrome, that no one really could explain, not even the doctors, is probably the most humiliating experience a person can live through. As you can't help but feel that losing your active lifestyle and having to be bedridden, then being shamed on top of the illness is something that the public should know about, whether they struggle or not! A patient with ME/CFS can feel as if they are actually losing their minds. No wonder they referred to those in Iceland as suffering with what they thought was "hysteria" you try waking up one day and being so exhausted, and that exhaustion never goes away. After you gain 8 hours of sleep or 10 hours, or sleep for even 12 hours, you never feel refreshed or rested. It's difficult to be 'normal' when life as you knew it is now gone.

Perhaps I sound negative, but that is entirely too long for anyone to suffer with a disease in this country and it not being recognized. Entirely too long. Now, what is more shocking? That it is now 2019 as I write this to the public there is still no know pharmaceutical medication that can counteract these symptoms, nor is there a cure.

Now let us explore M.E. on Wikipedia and how they tied the two ME and CFS together. Many medical websites may even say that M.E. is Chronic Fatigue Syndrome and vice versa. Yet most that struggle will tell you that they do feel different at times. Looking at just CFS, because back in the mid-eighties M.E. or Myalgic encephalomyelitis wasn't spoken about that I'm aware. 'Chronic Fatigue Syndrome' or CFS was identified as the "Yuppie disease."

One day I realized that we as a community of people with Chronic Illnesses, needed a mode to connect to people without Invisible Illnesses. There became an obsession in our own fibro support group to find people who would like to write to spread awareness. Our format is easy for any reader to enjoy at age 18 and over. Reading this book, anytime of the day, where a reader can feel comfortable and not judged. This became an obsession as I took a break from creative fiction writing to put these books together and a team of excellent people joined forces and Invisible Publications was born. I certainly wasn't a publishing expert, but I knew how to self-publish and I knew a few office skills necessary to put the collaborations together. The passion came from caring, when you believe in an idea so strongly as it will give others healing and validation, hiring only those with invisible diseases.

Some people learning new self-publishing skills and learning writing skills and the apps that relate to this type of work. This is how entrepreneurs got their start in this world, by learning the necessary skills and to keep pushing forward. Since then our team has grown from one author to a few co-authors' as well as numerous interested writers helping to fill our pages. They may have a close family member that struggles. They may have a close friend or a partner, or a spouse that has been diagnosed with ME/CFS. They need this book just as much as those that are actual sufferers.

This is an important factor with our books. All writers are patients, or some may be a family member of a patient. We ask that the patients write their story in an email and send it to us. We do the rest. They do not pay a dime; in fact, they do receive minor incentives and opportunities to win prizes or join our company.

Most write because they want to get the word out. It's as simple as that.

As this debilitating disorder grows in numbers across the nation and the globe, our population also grows. That's the connection, who else, on this globe, goes through this on a daily basis, who else feels the isolation and to be honest who else feels demeaned by a business world that people must be alert and ready to tackle the largest problems quickly and in an efficient fashion. We lose our attention span at any time of the day, we can shut down and need to rest or to have something to eat to snap back.

We're not participating in these publications to sugar coat things. Oh no, none of these diseases, disorders or syndromes are fun at all. But we do believe that we heal by writing and we can have fun. In fact, one of our other recent publications was on the topic of enjoying a vacation with fibromyalgia. We need to laugh at ourselves and allow fun into our lives. All of us that work putting this book and other books together struggle with either this disorder or a similar disorder that is not only Invisible but has also changed their life.

My dream is that everyone can learn about these disorders and then the stigma starts to change. Chronic Pain does not have to be an embarrassment or a stigma if it affects your personality or your need for more medications than the average guy or gal. The stigma that comes with ME/CFS is that of someone who seems sick all the time, seems "out there," or you look so pale, why don't you get some sun. Our bodies can literally "shut down" when taxed. We watch our spoons just like a fibromyalgia patient, but in a different way. I watch for over activity more so than someone with just one disorder. I have double the trouble and double the fun, so I need to use 50% less spoons than perhaps someone with just fibromyalgia. Although, we each have our personal spoon count and only the patient themselves know what that is.

Each diagnosis is a blow to our ears as it is when we continue to live with each one's assault on the body. Each of us have the cluster affect (meaning that we struggle with more than one), M.E/CFS, fibromyalgia, Rheumatoid Arthritis, Reynaud's Syndrome and a slew of others. As I write this my thoughts go to Brooke Whipple, an upcoming co-author for our next book project. Her multiple illnesses and symptoms became overwhelming for her to handle while working on that upcoming book. One of us becoming ill, meant that it was possible upcoming book could become delayed.

Writers' depended on us to complete our efforts quickly as possible and get their stories published. The co-author for this book, Donna Short RN, stepped up to the plate to assist Brooke with not only the book's organization but the group participation and much more. Each of us struggle with invisible diseases. We are here working for you, working for the effort, working for validation for each and every one of us that struggle, and suffer each and every day with CFS or fibro.

To watch one team member, help another team member, when they too are struggling is very touching. To watch our co-authors and writers, pray for our team members, as we went through our own struggles while putting the various projects together. Writing an introduction to one of our books is something I delight in, putting my thumbprint here for each of you to enjoy is rewarding. Allowing you to know me, and by reading our other titles you will find I'm very open. I will no longer hide my truths. Yet it had been so long since I felt the horrid symptoms of my recent flare, it was actually a blessing in disguise. Yes, I said that! It was a blessing! Let me explain. Believe it or not, those awful symptoms that had just escalated bringing the pain and exhaustion to the forefront of my memory, giving me the inspiration to get this introduction completed.

Donna Short R.N. the co-author of this title is an amazing and accomplished woman. Our partnership has been extremely rewarding as she wants to bring you the best possible publication. Organized and dedicated, it's been a pleasure to work with her on this project and our future books as well. We have other books titles on the back burner, and we don't know where this will take us all. One thing for sure our days are never boring with team comradery and cheering each other's books towards completion.

For myself, since I can't speak for the rest of the publishing team it's been a dream come true. They say "find a job you love, and you'll never work again" is how I want everyone to feel that contributes one or many stories to Invisible Publications. Whether it's a like on our page, a comment in one of our groups, a review on amazon, whatever your participation, we hope you enjoy taking part in what we are doing.

If you have this horrid illness, I applaud you for reading this book. You need to know you are not alone. If you feel a connection with this 4th book in our series, I do hope you reach out to us and let us know what you thought of our stories. We want you to know that we are here for you, either by email or by messenger. Join our groups and meet us, we welcome you with open arms!

Help us spread awareness by telling others about our titles as we depend on word of mouth. We did this for you, for all that struggle and all that want to learn about how our invisible illness affects our day to day lives. Now we will ask you to be there for us. If you are a fan of the publication(s) we need your help to spread awareness. Ask your library to carry our publications, this can usually be done right online with your county libraries. Share our book links on Social Media. Perhaps you too have a story to tell. We are looking for stories for our future publications. You can find out more with our Facebook page and our website.

Everyone is valuable. You are the ME/CFS, you are a human being with so much to offer. Many of us that work on these books may be housebound, or even bedridden the majority of the time. We use our small netbooks and iPads, even our phones while resting in bed to get the word out. We may not be out in the workforce due to the complexities of holding a full-time job with this condition, but we will not let that stop us. Writing a few stories and then feeling a sense of healing is an amazing feeling! We have stories to tell and people who wish to hear them! Enjoy!

References:
Wikipedia.com

Mepedia.com

www.cfstreatmentguide.com/blog

I would like to dedicate this book to my Dad in Heaven, you always taught me to chase my dreams and you always said you can be anything you want to be with hard work and perseverance. You were right, I am an author now, I did it! I love you, see you soon! And to my Husband Tom, thank you for loving me through sickness and health. Thank you for all you did as we took care of my parents, and still to this day you continue to help me get through the sorrow of my broken heart.

I would also like to thank all the now published writers that were brave enough to come forward and put their heart and soul into their stories for you, our readers. I thank you for standing up and using your voice. This book would not be possible without all of you! You all have a special place in my heart as we all stand together to bring awareness of ME/CFS to the public. Much love and many blessings.

Susan Parker Rosen, I can't thank you enough or put into words how much gratitude I have for you giving me this opportunity! To many more to come! Much love my dear friend!

Donna Short RN

{16}

I dedicate this book to all the ones who are truly suffering, the ones who can't get out of bed, or can't walk, must have a caregiver, or live in a nursing home due to this terrible illness. I want you to know that I care, I understand, and I am your advocate and this book is your voice. Keep rising from the ashes and never give up hope. Never give up, and always try to see the beauty in everything. Don't concentrate on what you can't do, but keep your focus aimed at what you can do! You are the true heroes in this world, the ones that suffer daily and have no cure in site. Keep rising from the ashes and never give up hope. I hope to help change that for us one day and know that I am working hard for all of you. We are all in this together, and I won't stop fighting until my last breath.

Donna Short RN

Letter From the Author

By Author Donna Short RN from Michigan, USA

"Compassion literally means "to suffer together." The feeling that arises when you are confronted with another's suffering and feel motivated to relieve that suffering. Compassion is not the same as empathy or altruism, though the concepts are related. What the medical community and public needs to understand is that individuals suffering with an invisible illness need compassion, our world needs more compassion for those that suffer together." ~**Donna Short RN**

I chose to co-author this book because not only am I a ME/CFS warrior, I'm an advocate for those who don't have a voice. For the warriors that can't get out of bed, completely bed bound and now a burden to loved ones (at least that's what we think, or how we feel.) The ones that are really struggling, the severe cases. The medical field and the public doesn't understand the magnitude of this illness.

Those that can't finish brushing their teeth or finish a meal due to exhaustion. For those that can't stay awake or can't walk. For those trapped in four walls, or yet, the edges of their bed. The pain of atrophied muscles, severe muscle spasms, along with the loss of dignity, self-worth and lost purpose. Imagine this.... I really want you to put yourself in our shoes.... you become more exhausted over a period of about four months. You were perfectly fine before it started, you were working out, working and living life. Suddenly, you start missing a lot of work because you are so exhausted that you can barely use your phone to call in. Let's pause for a moment and talk about the true definition of exhaustion.

I believe that doctors and the public think that we are just tired or low on go-go juice, lazy even. No. How insulting! We didn't ask for this! Let's really put this into perspective. Let's look at the definition. According to collinsdictionary.com, "exhausted means the state of being so tired that you have no energy left". Now please, really sit with that for a moment and imagine what it would be like to have absolutely no energy left. Nothing. Like having a terrible flu, or the day after receiving chemotherapy. That type of exhausted.

Let's take a quick look at the real definition of energy. According to collinsdictionary.com, energy is the ability and strength to do active physical things and the feeling that you are full of physical power and life. Now please sit and think how you would feel if you were completely depleted of energy. Before you know it you're filing for FMLA, next your career is taken from you because you physically can't get up, clean up, get dressed, eat, and get into your car much less the building you work in, and you are not getting better. Now you are not working because you are not physically able.

The bills still need to be paid, you start becoming monetarily trapped and defeated, too tired to fight with your debtors and you end up losing your home or filing bankruptcy because you have no income coming in. Next thing you start to realize is that you now need someone to take care of you and everything else too! Simple tasks like, making a meal, taking the garbage out and taking care of the lawn. Now what? Please, understand that we are not seeking sympathy, or pain pills to get high, instead we are just desperate for some type of pain relief, or some type of answer! (Well it's true, that's what the public and doctors think!)

It's a stigma, and that's what we have come together to break! This book is our voice, our fight and it's your wakeup call! Our lives are so restricted to the very little that we can do, we feel useless, broken and unworthy. We honestly don't know what to do with our lives, lives filled with exhaustion and pain. These stories in this book are real, from real people, full of emotion and despair, they are raw, nothing to be held back. Some very sad. Writers pouring their hearts out on paper. Desperate for healing, we don't want to just exist, we want to live.

We want to be a productive part of society we want to work and provide and have our purpose back. We don't want to continue to be the millions missing out on life. We need compassion and understanding. (We are not going to take "It's all in your head." anymore! Nor a doctor telling us "I don't believe in ME/CFS, you're just depressed.") We are coming together, we have a voice, we are using these stories for awareness and education. We are judged so much, and it needs to stop! Stop sweeping us under the rug or getting us out of your office quickly because you have no answers.

We are people who just want help, we don't want to suffer anymore. Suffering that needs compassion. As a nurse I have done extensive research on ME/CFS which gives me the opportunity to put this book together and share what I have learned with all of you! What is ME/CFS? According to the CDC (Centers of Disease Control) "myalgic encephalomyelitis/chronic fatigue syndrome (ME/CFS) is a disabling and complex illness." People with ME/CFS are often not able to do their usual activities. At times, ME/CFS may confine them to bed.

People with ME/CFS have overwhelming fatigue that is not improved by rest. ME/CFS may get worse after any activity, whether it's physical or mental. This symptom is known as post-exertional malaise (PEM). Other symptoms can include problems with sleep, thinking and concentrating, pain, and dizziness. People with ME/CFS may not look ill.

However,

» People with ME/CFS are not able to function the same way they did before they became ill.

» ME/CFS changes people's ability to do daily tasks, like taking a shower or preparing a meal.

» ME/CFS often makes it hard to keep a job, go to school, and take part in family and social life.

» ME/CFS can last for years and sometimes leads to serious disability.

» At least one in four ME/CFS patients is bed-or house-bound for long periods during their illness.

Anyone can get ME/CFS. While most common in people between 40 and 60 years old, the illness affects children, adolescents, and adults of all ages. Among adults, women are affected more often than men. Whites are diagnosed more than other races and ethnicities. But many people with ME/CFS have not been diagnosed, especially among minorities.

There are;

>> An estimated 836,000 to 2.5 million Americans suffer from ME/CFS.

>> About 90 percent of people with ME/CFS have not been diagnosed.

>> ME/CFS costs the U.S. economy about $17 to $24 billion annually in medical bills and lost incomes. Some of the reasons that people with ME/CFS have not been diagnosed include limited access to healthcare and a lack of education about ME/CFS among healthcare providers.

>> Most medical schools in the United States do not have ME/CFS as part of their physician training.

>> The illness is often misunderstood and might not be taken seriously by some healthcare providers.

>> More education for doctors and nurses is urgently needed so they are prepared to provide timely diagnosis and appropriate care for patients. Researchers have not yet found what causes ME/CFS, and there are no specific laboratory tests to diagnose ME/CFS directly.

Therefore, doctors need to consider the diagnosis of ME/CFS based on in-depth evaluation of a person's symptoms and medical history. It is also important that doctors diagnose and treat any other conditions that can cause similar symptoms. Even though there is no cure for ME/CFS, some symptoms can be treated or managed. The symptoms of myalgic encephalomyelitis/chronic fatigue syndrome (ME/CFS) may appear like many other illnesses and there is no test to confirm ME/CFS. This makes ME/CFS difficult to diagnose. The illness can be unpredictable.

Symptoms may come and go, or there may be changes in how bad they are over time. A doctor should be able to distinguish ME/CFS from other illnesses by doing a thorough medical exam. This includes asking many questions about the patient's health history and current illness and asking about the symptoms to learn how often they occur, how bad they are, and how long they have lasted. It is also important for doctors to talk with patients about how the symptoms affect their lives. There is no cure or approved treatment for myalgic encephalomyelitis/chronic fatigue syndrome (ME/CFS).

However, some symptoms can be treated or managed. Treating these symptoms might provide relief for some patients with ME/CFS but not others. Other strategies, like learning new ways to manage activity, can also be helpful. Patients, their families, and healthcare providers need to work together to decide which symptom causes the most problems. This should be treated first. Patients, families, and healthcare providers should discuss the possible benefits and harms of any treatment plans, including medicines and other therapies.

Healthcare providers need to support their patients' families as they come to understand how to live with this illness. Providers and families should remember that this process might be hard on people with ME/CFS. I myself live with hypothyroidism, fibromyalgia, chronic fatigue syndrome and everything that goes along with it. I know what it feels like to lay in bed all day and all night because your physically weak. I was bedridden for three months, I had my career taken from me, friendships gone, socialization gone. It steals your goals, dreams and joy. It literally feels like the old you has died, and now you're left with a body that can do very little but a mind that wants to continue its purpose.

Post-exertional Malaise (PEM) Post-exertional malaise (PEM) is the worsening of symptoms after even minor physical, mental or emotional exertion. The symptoms typically get worse 12 to 48 hours after the activity and can last for days or even weeks. PEM can be addressed by activity management, also called pacing. The goal of pacing is to learn to balance rest and activity to avoid PEM flare-ups, which can be caused by exertion that patients with ME/CFS cannot tolerate. To do this, patients need to find their individual limits for mental and physical activity. Then they need to plan activity and rest to stay within these limits.

Some patients and doctors refer to staying within these limits as staying within the "energy envelope." The limits may be different for each patient. Keeping activity and symptom diaries may help patients find their personal limits, especially early in the illness. For some patients with ME/CFS, even daily chores and activities such as cleaning, preparing a meal, or taking a shower can be difficult and may need to be broken down into shorter, less strenuous pieces.

Rehabilitation specialists or exercise physiologists who know ME/CFS may help patients with adjusting to life with ME/CFS. Patients who have learned to listen to their bodies might benefit from carefully increasing exercise to improve fitness and avoid deconditioning. However, exercise is not a cure for ME/CFS. Patients with ME/CFS need to avoid 'push-and-crash' cycles through carefully managing activity. "Push-and-crash" cycles are when someone with ME/CFS is having a good day and tries to push to do more than they would normally attempt (do too much, crash, rest, start to feel a little better, do too much once again). This can then lead to a "crash" (worsening of ME/CFS symptoms).

Finding ways to make activities easier may be helpful, like sitting while doing the laundry or showering, taking frequent breaks, and dividing large tasks into smaller steps. Any activity or exercise plan for people with ME/CFS needs to be carefully designed with input from each patient. While vigorous aerobic exercise can be beneficial for many chronic illnesses, patients with ME/CFS do not tolerate such exercise routines. Standard exercise recommendations for healthy people can be harmful for patients with ME/CFS.

However, it is important that patients with ME/CFS undertake activities that they can tolerate, as described above. It has been an absolute joy working with the writers for this book! I am so proud of them and as a team we were able to bring you this amazing book. I have a passion for teaching, and I truly enjoyed guiding and teaching my writers. I had one writer tell me that I give her hope and am a true inspiration to her for doing this. She is so excited for this book to get out there and bring awareness to those that are truly suffering.

This collaboration of stories helps them tell their story and have a voice and therefore I chose to do this. It is a passion of mine to give those suffering a voice. I have been truly blessed with this opportunity,

I can't thank Susan Rosen Parker enough for her guidance, mission, passion and most of all her love and friendship. To my writers thank you for devoting your time and energy into this project.

The writers are the real heroes, life itself gets in the way, they don't feel good, they are pulled in many directions and yet they persevered to write to have their voice heard. All of us with a chronic illness are the best actors and actresses too, we all deserve a Grammy because we are so sick and weak, yet we put on a mask every day. A mask of being normal, just to be accepted, just to "fit" in.

We feel so alone and afraid in this big world we watch from our beds or couches as everyone goes about their normal day, we yearn to have that back again, or even for the first time in some cases. I hope these stories bring hope to those suffering, educate our doctors and bring awareness to those that call us "lazy", or tell us we "need to exercise more". The best one is, "you don't look sick!" Those are some of the most hurtful things you could say to someone with a chronic illness. We don't want pity, we just want to have validation, believe what we tell you. Its real.

We want to break the stigma that goes along with chronic illness. We fight every day to try to be normal. All we need is to hear someone say, "I believe you."

Love & many blessings,
Donna Short RN
References: Centers of Disease Control (CDC)

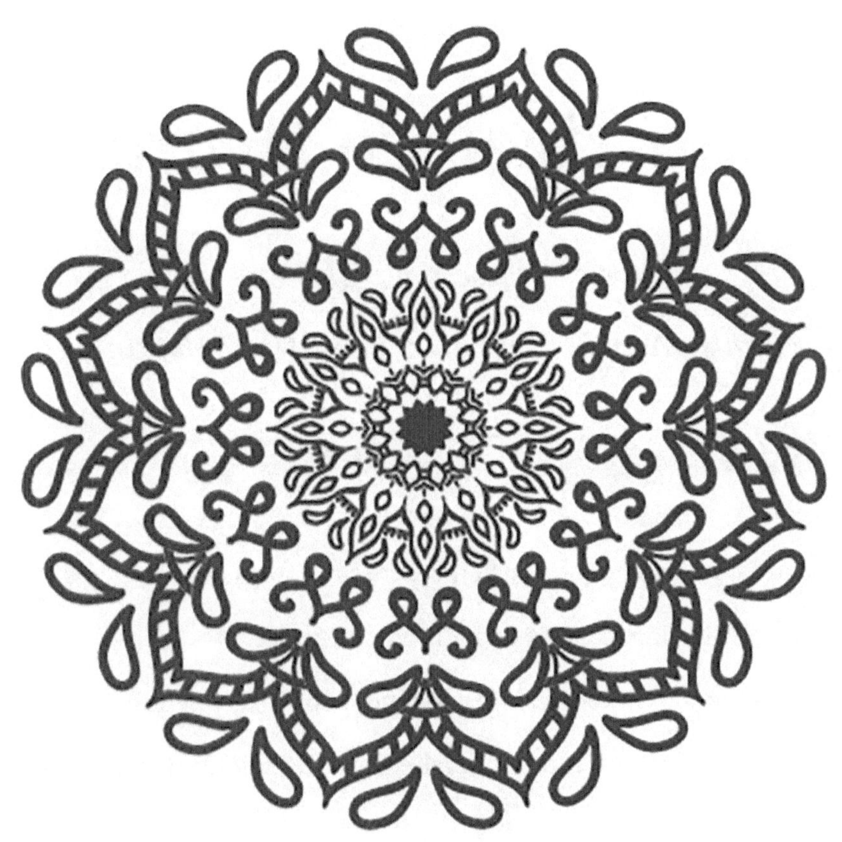

So Tired so Drained

Poem by Writer

Jenifairangel Goodman from West Virginia, USA

You know how you feel when you're tired from rain?

Imagine feeling like this with no time or frame.

Constant and never ending, good will people keep sending.

Rolling their eyes and so unbelieving, this feeling of being tired is so unsheathing.

Please let it go so I can keep going, everyone around me thinks I'm so annoying!

Day after day I keep telling myself, tomorrow I'll do better.

And then tomorrow comes and they all must settle.

I get tired of being tired and drained from being drained....

Can't I blame all of this on the unsettling rain?

My Drs, my kids, my friends, family and spouse, look at me like I am some kind mouse.

Because when they're all coming in, I choose to hide away in my den.

Too tired to talk, too tired to play, this constant fatigue needs just go away!

In the back of my head. I think one day it will.

But nobody believes me and all I can do is sit still.

So, with constant discomfort and too tired to go out.

I've lost all my friends and every youth outing they all sing about.

I wish I was me.... the me like before, climbing mountains and laughing and no dust on my floors.

So, with all this energy I've took.... I'm now off to bed.

See me now? Just look.

Famous
in My Fathers Eyes

By Writer

Asha Ryan from Ramsbottom, Lancashire, England

*"I don't need my name in lights, I'm famous in my Father's eyes
He knows my name."* ~**Francesca Battistelli**

Francesca Battistelli's latest worship song was playing quietly in the background, on the lounge stereo, when my husband came home from work surprisingly joyful after what is always a long day at the office for him. He leaned over to where I had been residing on the sofa for the past two weeks, to greet me with a kiss. Then he crouched down next to our daughter, Dee, who was playing merrily with her Legos on the living room floor. As she flung her arms around his neck in one of her scrumptious embraces, he wrapped his arms around her tiny waist and kissed her cheek. He asked what she had done at school that day. She replied with, "We learned about people who are different. Do you know Stephen Hawking?" "Yes" we replied in unison. "Do you know someone named Cox?" "No." We both said looking puzzled. Having racked our brains to think who she was talking about we finally gave up and I said, "Who is that?" "She's an athlete" said Dee." So, I Googled it on my phone. I found out it's Kedeena Cox, a world famous Paralympic. We also talked about Tom Cruise who has Dyslexia.

This was all very interesting you might think and so did I, but I felt this kind of weird feeling in my chest like an affront, a kind of indignation and I realized that I was angry. My husband and I looked at each other and he proceeded to explain to Dee, "These people are amazing, a bit like Mummy. She has CFS and she still manages to look after you and me, to make sure we have everything we need, get you to club on time and get you ready for school." My anger subsided thanks to the kind and unprompted acknowledgement from my husband, but it did leave me quietly questioning the wider issue.

Before I had M.E. I was a professional woman working in a corporate company, working my way up the career ladder. Then I got Glandular Fever. To cut a long story short, I didn't recover. I was spending 16 hours a day in bed. It would take me 3 hours to get up and get dressed, I couldn't cook meals, go shopping or socialize. Everything had changed. It has taken me 11 years to get to the stage now where I can function on a relatively normal level for 6 months of the year. The other 6 months I am in a flare up and predominantly housebound. Why are children in school being taught that someone with an illness is amazing only if they have overridden that illness and achieved great things? What about the rest of us?

Those who are missing from our previous lives, to take on the theme of #MillionsMissing? What about those of us who despite illness have not been celebrated on the world stage? Are we lesser people? Are we less significant? Am I less significant and less worthy of praise for my achievements because I haven't won any medals, or Oscar's? Are my sacrifices, my choices not good enough? Am I less important or valued less because I had to choose my health, my family and especially my daughter as my priority over a career and failing health? We are all fighting worthy battles in our private worlds and some of them are just as momentous as those that are being fought by the well-known and famous. Thankfully, as Francesca Battistelli says in her worship song, "I don't need my name in lights, I'm famous in my Father's eyes." You are too. I pray this gives each one of you comfort when you hear these stories that may dishearten you.

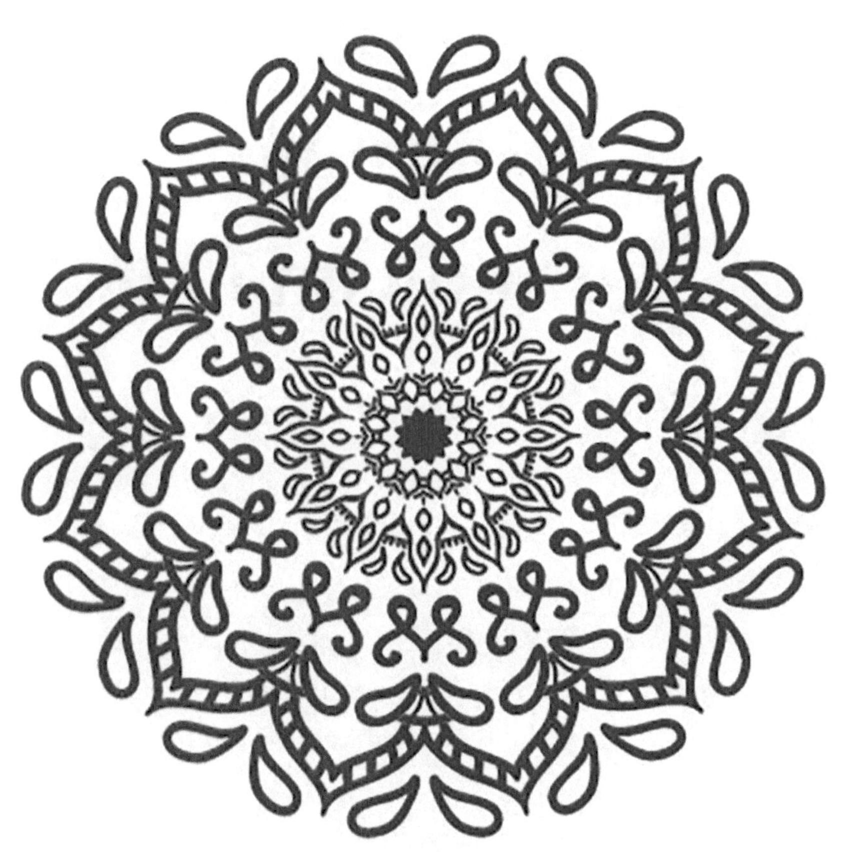

Chronic Fatigue and Me

By Writer Charmaine from Australia

"God grant me the SERENITY to accept the things I cannot change, the COURAGE to change the things I can, and the WISDOM to know the difference." ~Reinhold Niebuhr

According to Google dictionary:

Definition of Chronic:

"(of an illness) persisting for a long time or constantly recurring. A long-standing illness."

Definition of fatigue:

"extreme tiredness resulting from mental or physical exertion or illness."

The chronic fatigue I suffer with is from chronic fatigue syndrome. This can be debilitating by itself. Add fibromyalgia to the mix and this can make life an interesting adventure. You never know what the day will bring. Will I be able to get out of bed? Can I finish cleaning the house? Will I be able to function after visiting my mom who has Alzheimer's? These are some of the many questions I ask myself throughout the day.

I've had this for 12 years now (roughly). My life has changed from what you, the readers, would call normal, to a life that can change from hour to hour. Depending on the weather and what I did the day before. I'm always evaluating between what needs to be done and what I will be able to do, or the next day will be unproductive as my fatigue will be high. Somedays it's too high to even walk to the mailbox, which is only a few meters away.

My specialist wanted me to exercise to help with my fibromyalgia and chronic fatigue syndrome, mainly to prevent my muscles from wasting away. I was working at the time I was diagnosed. When exercise was mentioned, I couldn't imagine how I was going to be able to do exercise and work. So, I didn't do it. Working four days a week was enough for me at the time. Recovery after four days of work would take three days.

Concerned about the toll on my body and how I would cope with four days of work, I was guided by my GP to apply for the disability pension. The slow way was advised, taking nearly twelve months to achieve. I went from working four days to eight hours a week. I lasted around twelve months after receiving the pension, and then went to work only when they needed me. Eventually I left. It was just too much.

That was about four years ago. In those four years, I moved closer to my family and Mum, who was diagnosed with Alzheimer's. My daughter started three years of university doing midwifery. She had a five-year-old and a two-year-old, as well as a chief babysitter - me. This was a time where I learnt how to manage fatigue. Fortunately, this wasn't every day. Now, my daughter is finished and has graduated, working in a hospital close to home. I only do pickups from school and school holidays.

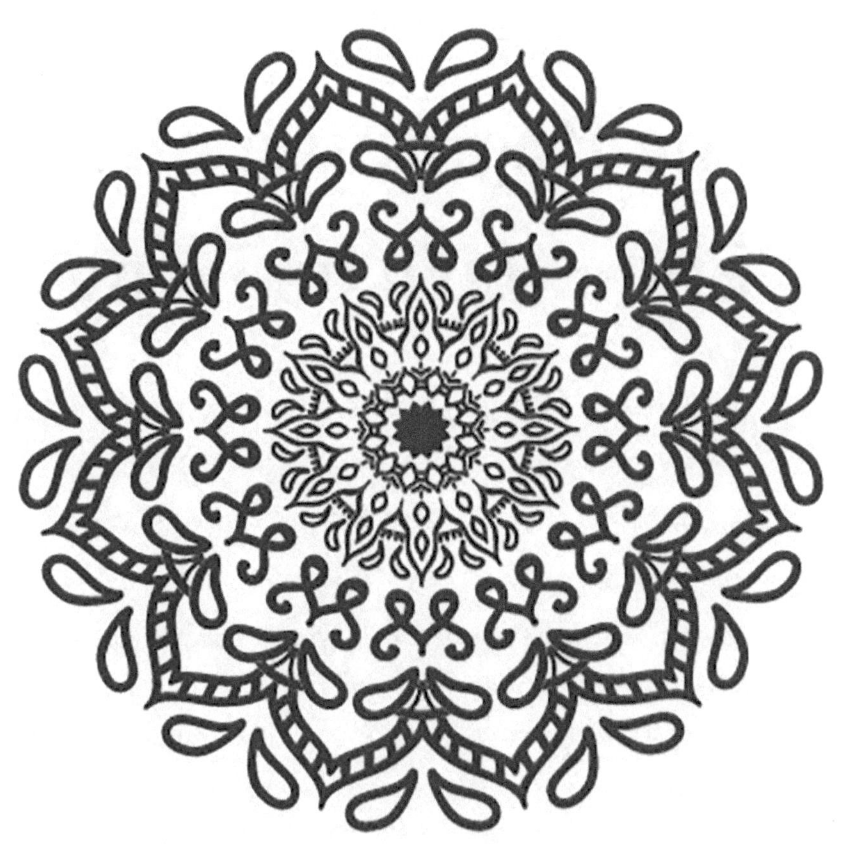

The Beginning of the End... Life as I Knew

By Writer Connie Jackson from Florida, USA

"Chronic fatigue syndrome can turn a life of productive activity into one of dependency and desolation... I have seen the horrors of this disease, multiplied by hundreds of patients." ~Jose Montoya, M.D.

I have written about the woes of pain in our previous books. After managing pain, undergoing major neck surgery, dislocated pelvis, and lots of physical therapy, God still gave me the ability to return to limited activities. I loved to garden, kayak, golf, lots of activities. But, sometime around 2013, my energy level started to go down. I found myself being tired all the time. Going to bed tired, waking up tired. I continued to have pain from my spinal conditions, degenerative disc disease, spinal stenosis, bulging disc, etc., etc., and the label of chronic fatigue syndrome. I didn't want to believe it, as I always thought it wasn't a true illness. That is, until I got it.

Sometimes I still do not want to accept this. But as you get diagnosed with autoimmune conditions; Sjogren's disease, psoriasis, thyroid issues, etc., etc., you start to think, maybe this is true. But not me! Then, the tiredness began to take over my life! I was getting too tired, so that I did not want to participate in outside activities.

Then it came to the point where I couldn't participate. At my worst, I didn't know how I was going to make it. I wasn't sure if I would be able to keep working. During this time frame, I had to go to the doctor every three months because of all the medications I was on. I began to tell my doctor that I was so tired. I was taking a diet pill for a while, but after losing the weight I needed to, he could not justify giving me the diet pill any longer. I begged him not to stop them because without them I couldn't function and didn't know if I would be able to get up. Again, I told him I was so tired! He wanted me to try another medication, which I did, and it helped somewhat, replacing the diet pill with another pill.

As days went on, my tired went way beyond the word for tired. I didn't know how to explain it. Where at one time I got up an hour early for my time with God and an hour early to walk before work, and be at work by 6:30, but now I was barely making it by 8:00, which was the time regular work started. I was a supervisor at the time, and it did not look good for me to be late for work every day. I was the type of person that wasn't late for anything. I was always early. Back to the doctor, again telling him I was so tired that all I could do was hurry and get home from work so I could lay down. That's all I did when I was not at work. Wake up tired, go to bed tired. I was not able to get up early. On workdays, I would get up and start to get ready for work; I would do one thing, then had to lay back down.

I would cry and pray, Lord, please help me to have the strength go get ready for work and get there. I would get up and do one other thing, then must go through that process several times every morning. At work, I had a yoga mat that I would put on my office floor during break and/or lunch. There were many times I would go in the restroom, pray and rest my head in my lap as long as I thought I could. I was also having increased pain. Back to the doctor again. This time, I told the doctor, I did not want to live anymore. I was not suicidal, but I didn't want to live life like that, barely able to get to work and couldn't wait to get home to lay down.

At that time, the doctor sent me to a hormone specialist. During all that testing, I did find out I had additional thyroid issues and hormones were out of whack. My lethargic state continued for some time. I did start to notice some difference. So much so, I met someone, married, and moved to Alabama in 2016. Due to the dating time and driving back and forth from AL to FL, I was somewhat concerned about my increasing neck pain. Where we were going to live was at least 30 minutes from town. After we came back from our honeymoon, I was already to the point I could not drive the 30 minutes and work with the pain I was in.

One month later, I had a thumb joint replacement. That put me in bed, started a severe CFS flare, and the severe fatigue started again. That was the beginning of another spiral in my health. One thumb surgery replacement in 2016, the other in 2017, pneumonia, and moving to a new location from Alabama to Florida. The move put me in to another CFS flare. I stayed in bed a lot. The fatigue was so bad, I would have to make choices of what I could do and what I couldn't do. You hear about the spoonie theory, you are given so many spoons for the day and each activity you do takes a certain number of spoons and once you use all your spoons, you were done for the day. I could relate!

Some days, it was literally all I could do to take a shower. I did not have the strength to wash my hair every day. I was not able to make meals. It was a chore to even make a sandwich. I thank God for giving me a wonderful husband! He has been so patient and understanding, trying to read up on the CFS conditions. He has been so loving through all my ups and downs. Thank you honey. I thank God that I have improved in a lot of ways. I still have to spend time in bed a lot during the day and fighting pain every day. But I can also stay up more than I have the last three years.

God has given me the ability to create crafts and turn a hobby into a business. I can only do a little at a time. Sometimes, I spend longer than I should, and my body pays for it. So, I really must pace myself; a few minutes here and there, resting in between. By the afternoon, I usually have to go to bed and some days I just must rest. I'm hopeful that things will improve.

Fatigued Beyond Belief

By Author Donna Short RN from Michigan, USA

"Courage is not having the strength to go on; it's going on when you don't have the strength." ~Theodore Roosevelt

I was diagnosed with CFS about a year after my fibromyalgia diagnosis. I remember sitting and doing paperwork and from my elbow down to the tips of my fingers felt like rubber and started burning. It was as if I was lifting a weight much heavier than I could obviously handle. I didn't understand what was causing this, I hadn't experienced this to this degree before. I would write for a bit, then I had to stop and wait for the burning and weakness to subside before I could start again. After a couple weeks of this I realized that my paperwork wasn't getting done on time which was not acceptable to Medicare. I was falling behind, and writing continued to become harder with longer breaks to not being able to read my writing at all. To this day my handwriting is not as good as it once was.

I also started to notice that while I was eating, usually at dinner time, my jaw was becoming tired from chewing. I had to soon start taking what I call "chewing breaks". Chewing breaks, is best described as: it feels like when you are chewing very tough meat and your jaw becomes tired, except it didn't matter what I ate. This was also continuing to become more difficult each day. My food was cold by the time I could finish my meal, I was always the last one to leave the dinner table. After I realized I was sitting there alone for a half hour after everyone else, I began feeling frustrated. It was getting harder and harder to sit at the table in a kitchen chair. I noticed my back muscles were starting to tire, and I began to have back spasms. I now eat in the living room in my rocker recliner.

Sleep, sleep, sleep. All I wanted to do was sleep. Often, I didn't have a choice and had to go to bed and sleep the rest of the day. I never wake up feeling rested and I will never know what it feels like to have that feeling again. CFS has stolen that from me, just like a thief in the night, taking all my energy restoring sleep. It is very sad and depressing. It's one of the hardest things for me to deal with. Imagine, never feeling rested, never feeling energized, never having energy to do anything. Every day I had to push and make myself do everything. I was weary, couldn't think clearly. Processing thoughts and coming up with answers were also becoming delayed.

Showers are exhausting, all the scrubbing and washing my hair was taxing. Toweling off was another process of stop, wait, dry off, stop, wait, dry off and the cycle continued. It took twice the time and energy to shower and get dressed; I would then have to rest afterwards. I would get up and make something to eat on a stool, do dishes from a stool and clean from a stool or sit on the floor Indian style because my legs had the feeling of burning and exhaustion. My legs even started to buckle under me, and I would fall. If I was unable to get up on my own, I would rest for a bit, then crawl to the couch. I felt as though my whole world was falling apart, my body was failing, I was becoming useless and a burden. This is even more debilitating, more devastating, slowly taking away the life I once had. The emotional pain is overwhelming and often unbearable, but I keep putting one foot in front of the other because I will never give up the fight.

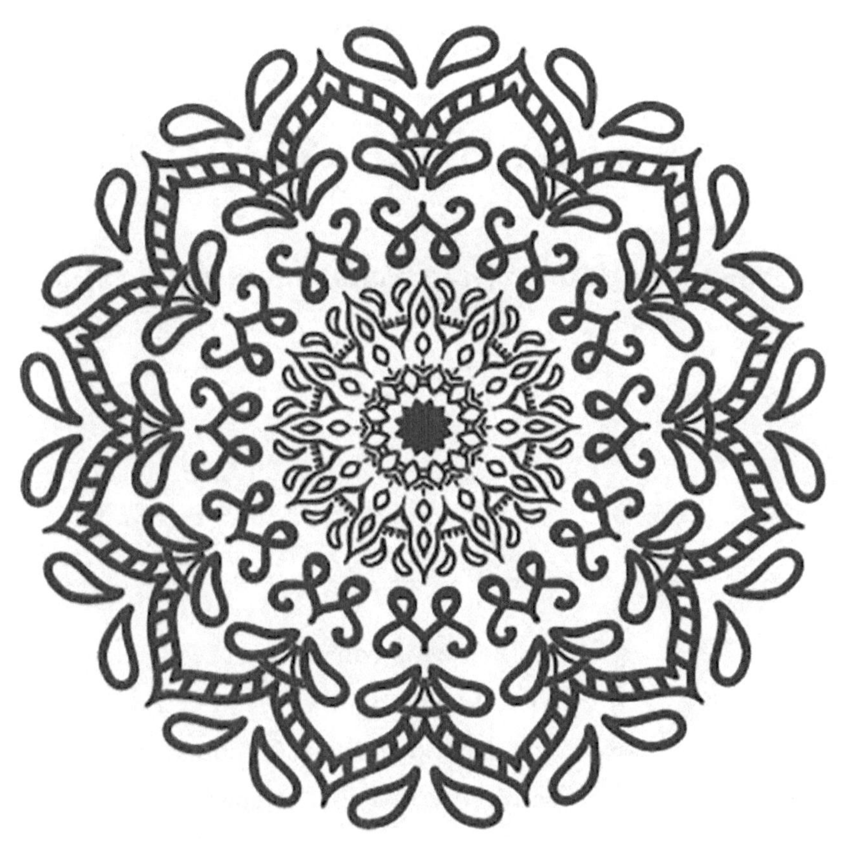

Hysterical Strength

By Author Jeanne Getz Pallos from California, USA

*Hysterical strength is a display of extreme strength
by humans, beyond what is believed to be normal. (Wikipedia)*

"Mom, I'm having contractions every twenty minutes. Can you come right away?" I could hear the panic in my daughter's voice. Of course, I'd go. Isn't that what mothers do? We dig deep to find strength we don't naturally have. Her husband had just started a job 160 miles away and would commute home on weekends. I was the only person she could call to watch her two-year-old toddler, my only grandchild, while she went to the hospital to get checked. As soon as I arrived, she headed for the door. "I'm sure it's nothing," she said. She even drove herself to the hospital, minutes from their home.

The baby wasn't due for two more months. We were still trying to figure out all the details for the birth. What if she went into labor while her husband was two hours away? Should they induce labor? Would I have the strength to watch my granddaughter and help my daughter with a newborn? Could I help them with the move after the birth? (She planned to stay in their home until the baby came. Then, she'd join her husband in a new city.) Anxiety had overwhelmed me every time I thought about the birth. Hopefully, they'd only need me for a couple of weeks. My worries were real.

After my daughter's wedding five years earlier, I'd spent months in bed recovering. After the birth of her first child, I collapsed for weeks. Each time, I pushed myself to the limit, praying that I'd have the strength to get through. I had struggled with chronic fatigue syndrome long before my daughter's birth in 1978. Before it had a name or recognition. When my daughter grew into her teens, she resented my limitations. Later, she told me, "You were always sick. You were never there for me." Her words haunted me. Now, I gathered every ounce of my strength to be the mother she needed me to be. As I fed and dressed my granddaughter, the phone rang. "Mom, I'm three centimeters dilated and in labor. They can't stop the contractions."

My husband rushed to the hospital, and my daughter's husband started the long drive home. I pressed my head against the wall and prayed. No matter my limitations, my daughter needed me.

The baby arrived at 8:20 p.m. and was rushed to the NICU (Neonatal Intensive Care Unit). I played with my granddaughter and tucked her into bed as if nothing was happening. My job was to keep her secure, safe, and happy. Could I do this? I had no choice. My daughter came home a few days later, without her baby. Her husband went back to work and I moved in with my daughter. While she visited the baby six hours each day, I cooked, did laundry, and entertained my granddaughter. We went for long walks, gathered leaves, created new games, and knit our hearts together.

Each night I collapsed into bed wondering how I'd make it through another day. And another. We had no idea when the baby would come home. I called my husband crying, "I can't keep going." But I did. The baby came home seven weeks later, but we delayed the move for another month. The pediatrician wanted to be sure he was stable. Inwardly I groaned. Another month. I can't do this. But I did. I spent three months living with my daughter and doing things far beyond my capacity. My daughter needed me. CFS couldn't stop me.

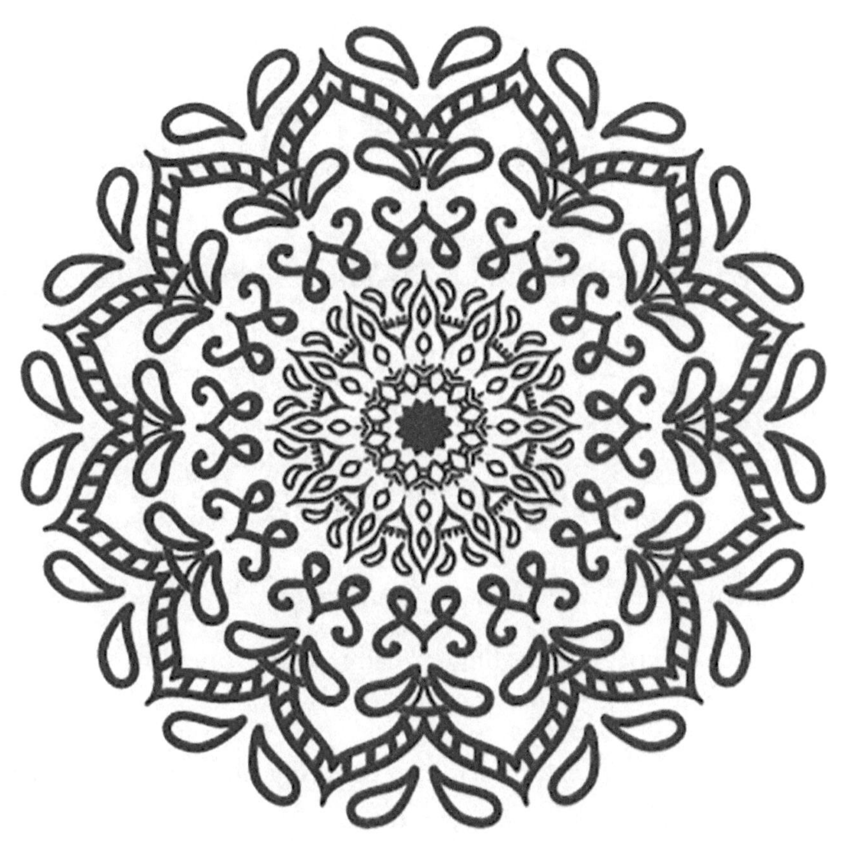

I'm Still Here

Poem by Jennifer Bartholomew from Illinois, USA

I AM NOT DISPOSABLE!!

Yes, I am different, my body, my mind twisted by disease

ravished with pain, struggling to maintain the appearance of being able bodied

sometimes I even trick myself into believing nothing's wrong, I'm just like I used to be, just like everybody else

then I push too hard and my brokenness shines like the wheels on my chair, like the metal on my cane

one day I woke up sick and I never got better, doctors were baffled, I was an enigma, a medical mystery

but I am still me, I am still here

no running by the lake anymore, no Zumba, no dancing till I kicked off my heels, stationary, secondary discarded by those who couldn't handle watching as the illnesses took control, seeing the pain proved too intense

as my friends skipped away, thoughts of what now lingered, deeply craving them to stay

often, I look up and whisper, "does anyone know I'm still here? my body is different, my mind is weaker

but I'm still ME... I still matter

I'M STILL HERE!!!

A Slow Fade

By Author Abby Guss from Ohio, USA

"I can and I will. ~Carrie Green

I have always been active, whether that is playing sports, spin class, personal trainers or lifting. I have always also battled with my weight, depression and anxiety. Some would look at my body and think it was great! But for me, I couldn't eat like other people. If I ate a dessert, I knew I would immediately gain some weight, get bloated or breakout. Since my mid-20s I noticed an issue with my blood sugar. I am not diabetic, but type 2 does run in my family. I was diagnosed hypoglycemic. Do you know the treatment for that? There isn't one! You basically suffer through it. Make sure you eat is what they tell you. I have been to countless doctors, and not one could tell me what to eat, when or why. I was over prescribed antidepressants, and my body was ravaged with pharmaceutical side effects like; constant weight gain, additional depression, and suicidal ideation.

At around 32 I noticed a significant change and a decline in energy, something was definitely wrong. People always say it's harder as you get older, but 32? I couldn't lose weight, no matter how well I ate or worked out. I was given even more antidepressants, which only made me gain weight and be more depressed, again. I couldn't take it and stopped them. The fatigue was a smidge better. At around 37 I noticed my energy level would bottom out. I was running 5K races, weight training, attending spin classes, and eating the appropriate number of calories. I should have been losing weight. I should have felt better and healthier.

At around 38 I began almost losing consciousness when my blood sugar would randomly drop. Then came on a panic attack. It felt like I was scrambling to survive. It would drop after eating also. By 40, I went from races, multiple spin & yoga classes, miles ran and lifting in the gym, to crawling up the stairs, inability to walk far, and then bed bound for a few months. It was during this time that my relationship also ended. I am sure it is hard to be with someone with an autoimmune or to them an invisible illness. It's even harder living with one.

The laundry list of commonality tells me we have reached an epidemic in medicine. Depression, panic attacks, anxiety, massive brain fog, inability to remember, lack of focus and concentration, insulin resistance, candida, blood disorders, fatigue, energy loss.....the only common thing I am seeing in my research is the consistency of symptoms people have, and lack of treatment for them.

I have traveled far, seen many doctors, specialists and those who love to call themselves functional medicine specialists. Many are snake oil salesmen, and at this stage I am unwilling to spend thousands more on doctors who give up after two visits.

I have tried elimination diets, organic everything, and seemingly every supplement available. While I still believe food can help a lot, I know other illness remains. I am currently treating myself.

I wish I could tell you I have conquered this, but it is a chronic illness. I am still struggling with daily fatigue, constant rosacea, gut issues no matter how hard I try, brain fog, bloating, weight problems and excessive fatigue. I miss my life. I miss my body feeling healthy, and I miss who I used to be. God willing, I keep trying every single day, and I won't punish myself anymore. I make sure I love myself every day as I am, and with that practice, I plan to get my health, mojo and life back.

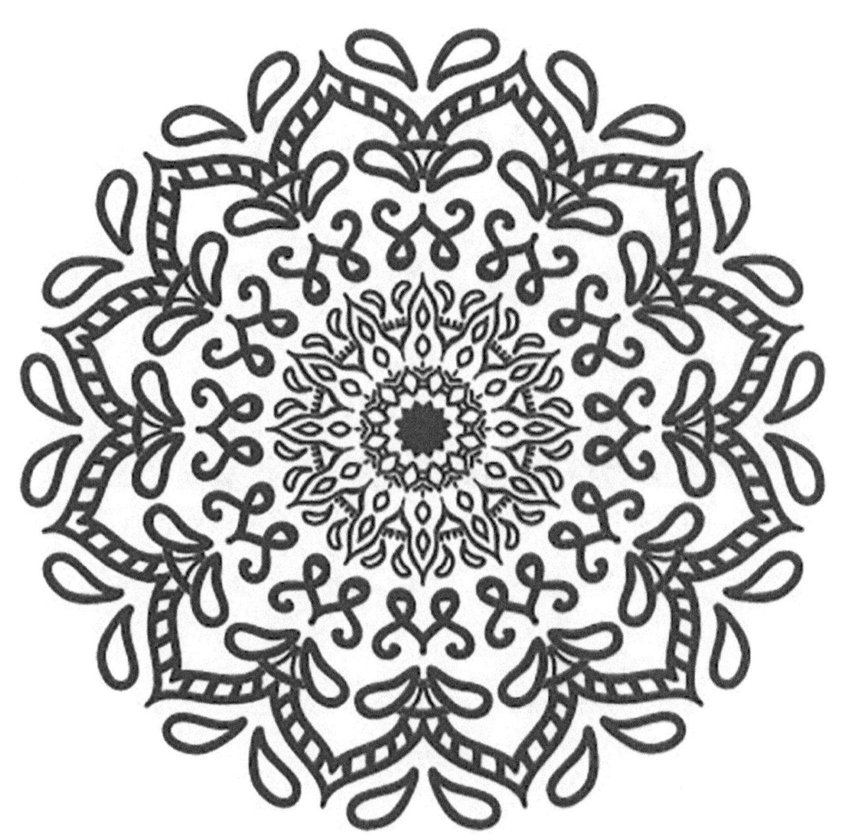

How My Suffering Days Go

By Writer
Deborah Denise Lafeber Macias from Texas, USA

"To live is to suffer, to survive is to find some meaning in the suffering."
~Friedrich Nietzsche

While my days start out like everyone else's by waking up in the early morning hours, I am dealing with my eyes burning and hurting because they are still so very sleepy. It's as if my body is also still very tired, like a nagging major fatigued tired feeling, as though I just never did rest and have had around six hours of sleep at least. So many nights it's way less and some nights more, it all depends on my mood and my difficult body, I guess. I literally lay there for a long while stretching and opening my eyes and blinking repeatedly thinking, "Ugh I really hate mornings and having to wake up because of my eye pains and my achingly stiff joints, muscles, ligaments, and tendons. It really hurts so much to even get out of bed, stand and walk.

Oh my goodness gracious I feel like I'm eighty years old already, because I have to literally force my mind and body every morning to function so I can just get up out of bed and go to the restroom, since that is obviously a must with nature ha-ha... It just really doesn't matter how much I try to rest and sleep because I still must struggle with being so very tired and constantly yawning all day long. It makes me wonder what I can change or do different to better myself and my everyday life. Oh man that just opened up a whole lotta mess for me, and of course it just depressed me more because I just don't have the energy to do much of anything else on top of what I already do as a single Momma, and as life in general gets in my way.

You know what is so very sad to me and really depressing is that I know that I am supposed to immediately thank our precious dear Lord God for even waking me up again and giving me another new day... I sadly am not thinking of being grateful to God at the very moment when I wake up every morning, mostly because I feel so very miserable: nauseous, dizzy, sick feeling, and I usually wake up with a major headache of some sort like a tension, cluster, or stress headache, or just an annoying horrible migraine. I'm still just so very tired that I feel hopeless and miserable because I've been dealing with this for like fifteen years or more. But hey, don't get me wrong here, because I am so very grateful to Jesus Christ for everything in my life, even though I don't always have the best perspective. Although my life is hard, I eventually realize that God is always working things out for my good, in His time of course.

I am often wondering why I must suffer with literally everything in my life, especially my mental and physical health, along with other hard things in my life, but then I think, "Who am I to question God?" I just have to thank Him for being there with me and holding me up, carrying me most of the time, because I feel in my heart that God is truly the only one that sincerely loves and cares for me, and is the only one that will never hurt me or disappoint me... I say all of that about our Lord because I believe that He is the only one that allows me to really deal with all the mental and physical illnesses. Illnesses that are invisible to most people prevent them from having a heart of understanding, compassion, empathy, or sympathy for people in the same situation as me.

It's a huge struggle and very lonely to be suffering in this way when others don't understand. It would feel a little easier if I visibly looked like something was wrong with me - like if I'd been injured or broke a bone. Honestly though, even when I was visibly suffering, it appeared that people were uncaring even then. I get looks daily when I park in the handicap spaces with my placard. When I get out of the car, I can see that they're wondering what's wrong with me. They don't see the things that I feel inside, or how difficult it is to walk after I've been grocery shopping. Everything I do just causes so much pain and tires me out so easily.

I know that through everything that I am currently suffering, and all that I have already been through, it has shown me that I am a survivor - an overcomer and obviously a persistent fighter. I guess I always have been, but I also have literally given up a few times and hit the very lowest rock bottom. I came to realize the hard way that I had to get back up and fight through all my struggles, even though I must suffer my way out of all the anguish I experience in this life.

I've been told more than once from different people that God obviously still has me here for a reason and He must have huge plans for my future and a better life... So, the main way I deal with all my struggles is in spending alone time with God in prayer daily.

Back in the 80s

By Author Susan Parker Rosen from Maryland, USA

"It is not the bruises on the body that hurt. It is the wounds of the heart and the scars on the mind." ~**Aisha Mirza**

CFS, chronic fatigue syndrome is also now known as ME, or SEID. I can tell you about the first time that I knew I was sick, why I think I became sick, and what it means to be struck by this disorder/syndrome. I became sick in 1985. I was employed by a carpet company outside of a city I do not want to mention. They did most of the commercial work at that time and they also did a huge residential business in an affluent area. The owner of the company was abusive and encouraged others to be bullies towards other employees, unless he favored them of course. There were also sexual comments and innuendos. Nothing that you could put your finger on, just not appropriate, if that makes sense. He did this when no one could hear him.

I was constantly bullied, reminding me of my childhood school mates and it began to break my spirit in life. Should I have filed suit, yes, but there was no way to prove it unless someone else came forward. And no one else did. I mentioned it to a co-worker who clearly was afraid for her job, since she would discount his comments, if I dared repeat the abusive comments to her. Why did I tolerate this treatment? I had a mortgage and bills, I looked for work elsewhere but the job market was horrid at the time. Hey, it was the mid-80s, sexual abuse was just coming into its own. As an attractive female out in the workforce, I took a lot of that. But this was different, his abuse was more demeaning than it was a come-on. If that makes any sense?! After all, my generation first saw the ability for women to wear pants to work.

To top off the constant hyper-vigilance to ward off triggers of bad memories, I would constantly overwork and try to "prove" myself. Not knowing that this toxic workplace was taking me back to issues I experienced as a young teen. The anxiety I felt was over the top. The kicker? The showroom sat on a sunny highway, and the sun would flow in turning the showroom into a sunroom filled with Monsanto products. When I would go home each evening I reeked of carpet, need I say more? Now, at the same time I was experiencing marital trouble, tried to get pregnant many times and could not. I hated my work, and my husband was spending more and more time out of the house. He was never home, when I say never...I mean he literally just slept there. He also started to travel a lot. The beginning of the end was coming, and I didn't know it.

One day, I was totally exhausted. I couldn't get up out of bed. I would lay there and try to move. Do anything, dress...put on slippers...go down the steps to make coffee. It was insurmountable. That wasn't the only symptom. I had a sore throat and my glands everywhere were so tender that moving my neck was excruciating. I went to a doctor that I had been seeing close to our new home and they said they couldn't find anything. They tested me for mono and it was negative. I tried a second opinion; the results were the same. I decided to go back to a family doctor that my family all used. He looked right at me and said, "You have a bug." He ran an Epstein Barr and that's what he diagnosed. But he was able to nurse me back to health, and I was able to return to work after a couple of weeks, but life was never the same for years upon years.

My mom called me one day, she said that a family member found an article about a new disease that some "yuppies" (their words not mine) from out west were first diagnosed with. It was being identified as Chronic Fatigue Syndrome! It was for life she told me. As she read off the symptoms, I realized that they were describing me. Inside I cried, nothing in my life was going right. And now on top of everything, I have contracted some strange disorder or sickness and I'll never recover from it. Little did I know that it was about to get worse, a lot worse before it got any better. More info to come when you read some of my stories within this publication!

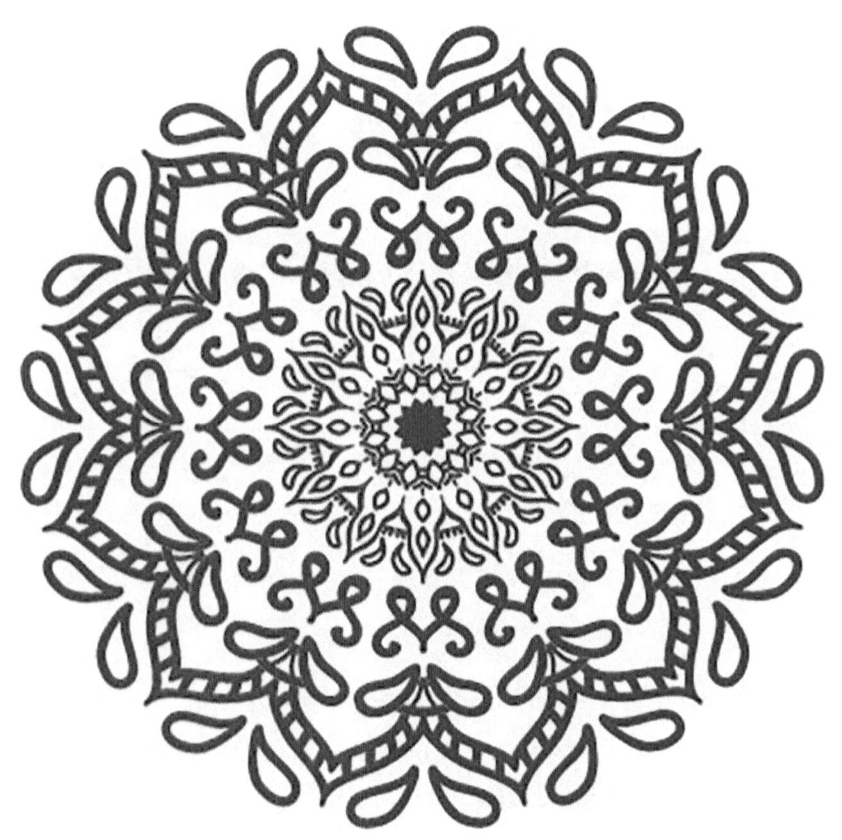

CF What?

By Author Robin Dix from Maine, USA

Ever since I hit menopause, I became very ill. Initially I was diagnosed with underactive thyroid and fibromyalgia. But within a few years it became very apparent that I was also suffering from chronic fatigue syndrome (CFS). Although I experience the pain associated with fibro, my fatigue has kept me mostly bed bound for over 6 years now. I've never been a high energy person anyway and I attributed that to having all my babies in my 30's. Who am I kidding, even as a teen and young adult I never had a lot of energy. For a long time though I didn't have a name for it, I thought it was something I was creating in my mind.

I think one of the hardest things about having CFS is dealing with family and friends who just don't get it. I can usually handle having company for about 2 hours or so, then I just MUST lay down. I have hit a wall and there is no energy left. When I get that tired it's difficult to think, never mind try to have a conversation. Rather than push through it though, I've learned to listen to, and honor my body. I'm the only one that will suffer if I push too hard.

I know that people mean well when they tell me I'd feel better if I exercised more. What they don't understand is that exertion of any kind for me results in PEM - post-exertional malaise. That means that, for example, when I take a shower, I need to lay down for hours afterwards to recover from that expenditure of energy. From the outside, it could appear that I'm being lazy, when I'm surviving.

CFS Is Not My Friend (Part I)

By Writer Candace Kay from Delaware, USA

"The world is more magical, less predictable, more autonomous, less controllable, more varied, less simple, more infinite, less knowable, more wonderfully troubling than we could have imagined being able to tolerate when we were young." ~James Hollis

I have had CFS as long as I can remember. Of course, when you are young, they just think you are lazy and unworthy. I wasn't lazy, I was tired! No one believed me and it was so frustrating. Knowing I was sick and no one else could see it. Mornings have always been the worse time of the day for me, I remember awaking and wanting to go right back to bed after breakfast. I did my duty of going to school and even though I was an honor student, I was partially comatose through classes I wasn't interested in. For example, why did I want to know about Ancient Chinese History? I'd come home from school, eat a snack, watch TV and fall asleep. I would wake up for supper, get a shower and do homework, and be in bed by the latest at 9, but usually it was before 8:30.

My mom had me tested for anemia and spoke to the family doctor on several occasions about what was making me so tired. The doctor could not find a diagnosis. He said it was probably me just growing too fast. Although my parents didn't complain much, I knew they were concerned, but my grades were good. I skated by in gym class by figuring out how many classes I could be out of without putting my grade in jeopardy. But why was I so tired? All. The. Dang. Time. The answers would come twenty-five years later.

CFS Is Not My Friend (Part II)

By Writer Candace Kay from Delaware, USA

"Start by doing what's necessary; then do what's possible; and suddenly you are doing the impossible." ~**Francis of Assisi**

Growing up I loved to read, do crafts and other things that people consider sedentary. Why? Because as a child I had every childhood disease and illness out there including whooping cough, chicken pox, and the measles. These diseases and illnesses compromised my immune system later down the road. My family always loved going to flea markets, car shows and auto races. These activities, as a teenager, wore me out halfway through the event we were at. Sometimes I slept on the way home.

Later in life, when I worked for a school district and had major holidays and summers off, I would spend my time occupying my kids or doing crafts or hobbies. My now ex-husband "suggested" I should be more productive outside like mowing the grass and gardening, and stop being "lazy." The heat and humidity zapped all the energy I had right out of me. How could I possibly be more productive by mowing the grass, if afterwards I wanted to sleep for 4 hours??? Well, that is not what the ex-hub wanted to hear. My chronic illnesses ended my marriage after 17 years.

After this incident I became known as the lazy wife with no energy. I had to delegate energy, according to the needs of the kids, cooking, and cleaning. That's enough to wipe a "spoonie" out. Energy conservation is so important for anyone with CFS or other chronic disease. One day or night of high energy can cost a "spoonie" days or weeks of recovery.

What is a "spoonie" you ask? That's a whole story within itself!

Where Is the House I Built?

By Writer Kari Ainslie from Ontario, Canada

"Fatigue is what we experience,
but it is what a match is to an atomic bomb." ~**Laura Hillenbran**

The other day, I was summarizing to my roommate how I have been feeling for the last few months. I told her that because my energy reservoir was so low, I was struggling to keep up with doing all the normal tasks of life. I kept waking up every day looking around to see if I could locate the house I built! I knew I had not actually built a house, but my energy had been so difficult to manage that my daily life that did not consist of employment at the time, felt strenuous enough that I compared it to the building of something grand. It is the strangest thing for me to tell you that this feeling is so new to me, and yet not new at all as I've been struggling with chronic illness since February 2015 (currently, that is for four years and four months). It was only in August 2018 that I received one of three of my diagnoses: chronic fatigue syndrome.

The easiest way to explain chronic fatigue syndrome to you is this: An average person goes to sleep, and it is like putting their phone on a charger. When they awake, their phone is 100% (or close to it) and they go about the day. A person with chronic fatigue syndrome does the same, except they wake up daily to find the phone charged only a minimal percentage, and that percentage is different each day. They then must go to manage their day on this minimal percentage without the phone dying.

It's not about waking up a bit tired, drinking some coffee, having a hot shower, and pushing yourself to feel more awake (or to endure). It's literally that you are so tired that every daily task expends energy. Every single task becomes a matter of pacing which can be a confusing, disappointing, discouraging, or frustrating process. When the phone is dead, a recharge must occur. If one pushes past that point, they are then borrowing charge from the next day and the next and maybe even the one after that. The recharge process will take even longer.

A person with chronic fatigue syndrome has so much to consider including how energy can be drained physically (standing, walking, cooking, cleaning, etc.), emotionally (going through a hard time, stress, etc.), and even mentally (reading a book, engaging in a conversation, etc.). They have environmental considerations that affect energy that are probably just "background noise" to a normal person such as: lighting, noise, smells, amount of people in a space, etc.

Even simple tasks become an effort that can require extreme concentration. It can also be difficult to feel present in a moment, if I feel like I am not fully awake! I've found that pacing myself is the most important thing I can do. I've also found that when I don't listen to my body and I push, I get worse. As I mentioned, this feeling is not new to me, but the name of it and official diagnosis is. Before I was diagnosed, I journaled on March 11, 2018, and this is how I described it:

"I honestly just feel so sick! I honestly just want to get better, get well. Sometimes it just feels like I'm getting nowhere. It's like when you're peddling your bike on the wrong setting and you are turning the pedals over and over so many times, but the bike only actually moves like a tiny bit of ground. I think how my heart's cry repeatedly has been to stop trying and rest. To put the bike away in the garage and spend some time fixing the gears instead of trying to ride it broken! My heart's cry has been to heal, and then to get on the bike."

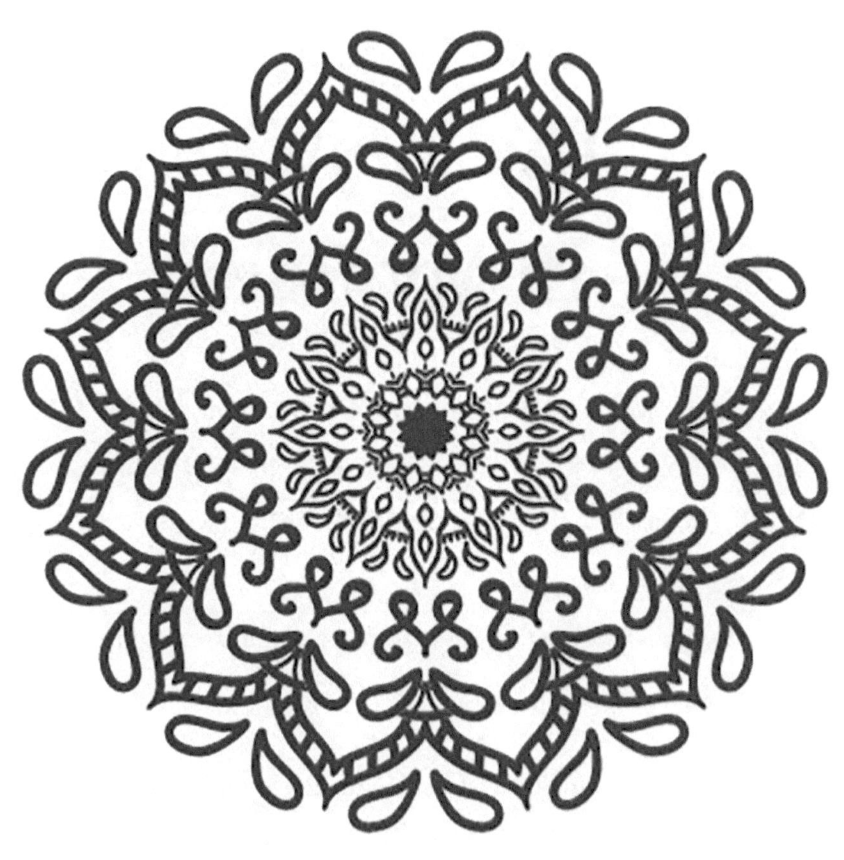

The Monster in My Body

By Writer Deborah Walenta from Texas, USA

"You never know how strong you are until you have no other choice."
~Unknown

I've had two major car accidents in my life, one in 1984 and another in 1990. Then in 1992, while in my first trimester of pregnancy I was injured on the job. It took another 11 months after my daughter was born that the doctors, colleagues, and friends believed me. Three back surgeries later, I'm left with chronic lower back pain, and nerve damage down my right sciatic nerve to my leg.

Welcome Monster #1.

One morning in the middle of the 90's, I'm sure that's when my other Monsters came to life. No one knew what to call all my aches and severe pain and exhaustion. I was labeled a hypochondriac by doctors and friends. My husband even questioned my sanity. The Monsters, 2 & 3 had moved into my body and decided they LOVED it so much, they weren't EVER GOING TO LEAVE! Monster #2 is my Fibromyalgia, but that story is for another day and time. And boy is it a doozy.

I'm going to tell you my story with CFS, Aka Monster #3. If you have CFS, it's going to sound familiar, if you don't have CFS hopefully you will understand more once you pick up this book. My CFS started off slow and I honestly thought it was my Fibro being a jerk. I started writing down all my symptoms. Severe exhaustion; like I had been running for a week straight with no break. Realizing there's no fuel left in "my" tank.

Forgetting words; I'll be in the middle of a conversation and suddenly, I'm at a loss for words and can't remember what I was saying. God forbid if I'm talking and someone or something breaks my concentration, I won't remember what I was saying before the interruption- it's all gone. Or if I'm talking and the words won't come out correctly. I know what I want to say, but I can't articulate the words. For example, I'm telling my daughter about the day I had with my grandson. I wanted to tell her about his walker, but I couldn't get the words out no matter how much I tried. She didn't understand me and so I had to point to the truck to show her what I meant. It's embarrassing and frustrating all at the same time.

I wake up so very tired. I could sleep all day and still not feel energized. I must watch how much energy I expend every day, because if I ever do everything. I end up "paying" for it later or the next day by being in a lot of pain and exhausted, and only wanting to be in bed. There are times that even the air flow from a fan or the AC, hurts my skin. Dirt on my sheets can feel like glass on my body. Any weight can feel like boulders when my body is in a flare. We desperately want to be hugged. We need a connection to others, but our bodies hurt. So even a hug can send someone into a spasm. My Lymph Nodes are swollen like others, mine just happens to be in my neck and are painful to the touch. I've had that pain for over 20 years.

That's something I wouldn't wish on my worst enemy. I've already lived with all this pain, and exhaustion since I was 26, and now I'm 54. Since then I've lost friends throughout the years, and I still don't have anyone I can talk to in person. I have my support groups, but it's not the same. So...no pity party I seriously doubt there will be a cure for CFS in my lifetime. But it IS one of the Invisible Diseases, and what the public doesn't realize is that you can die from CFS. By the Grace of God, I won't die by one of my Monsters.

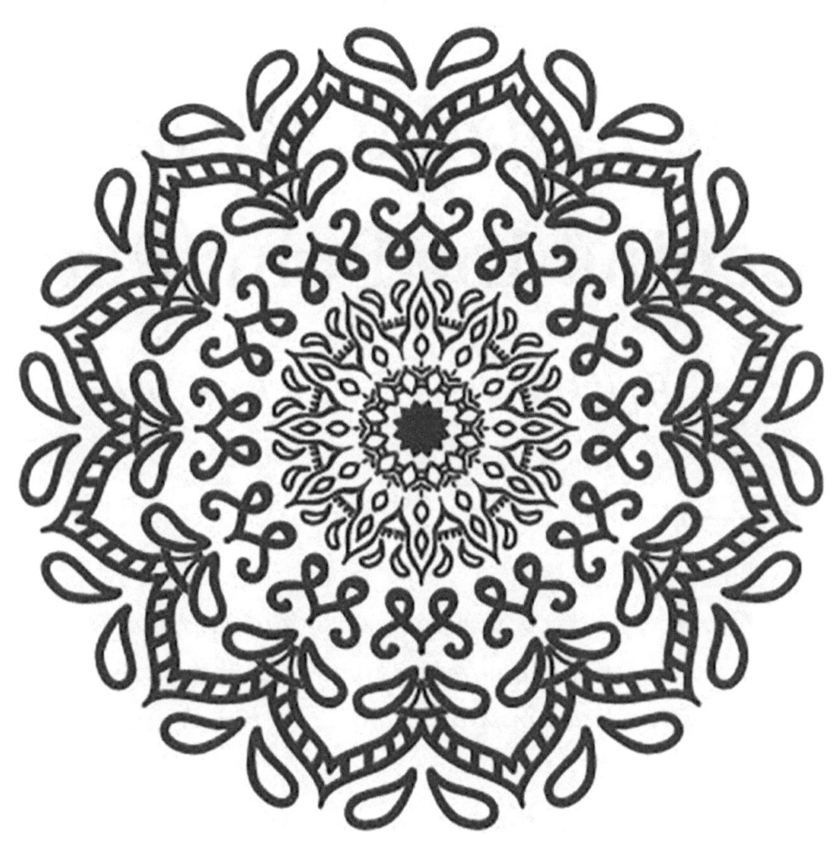

The Invisible Blessings Behind the Pain (Part 1)

By Writer Gargi Sanyal from India

Character cannot be developed in ease and quiet. Only through experience of trial and suffering can the soul be strengthened, vision cleared, ambition inspired, and success achieved. ~**Helen Keller**

It was 9pm sharp, the storm was just over. At 5-yrs old little Binnu was merrily playing with her Barbie doll in her room now, as her Meme had arrived home a couple of hours after attending her doctor's visit. It was a hectic journey and a long day of exhaustion, so Mamma was resting in her bedroom since she returned to overcome her tiredness. 10-yr old Tinnu, being a bit mature, was unable to play freely knowing her Mama's anxiousness about the doctor's opinion today regarding her disease which was not getting any better for more than 5-yrs! Being worried, Tinnu silently went to her Mom's room and took out the medical documents from her bag to find out about her illness.

Suddenly, a small diary fell from her hand named 'Brief history by Gargi'. Tinnu started reading it: "I belong to a Middleclass-Bengali-Hindu-Indian-Nuclear-family with only one elder brother of mine. And then there's society! It was such that it followed, also imposed in most of its level ill practices of male patriarchism, being continued even today. Since childhood, I bear a highly sensitive and moral character and overall a good performer. Thus, though not educationally or financially solely, but my upbringing was done, in not at all an emotionally content way, rather it occurred in an emotionally low environment both in house and socially!

As per medical history is concerned my father has rheumatoid arthritis, mother is a patient of hypertension, and myself, bronchial asthma. That's all! At 22, I got married which was a partly arranged one as we knew each other just for some days beforehand. With God's grace I was blessed with my two beautiful daughters during the period of my rise and plateau like married life, which is finally over now!! Presently my family means me and my two daughters, who are my only world. Legal cases are on and worst of all I needed to quit my job too, and am on work-from-home jobs for flexible timings, to overcome my symptoms such as; regular fatigue, muscle pain, severe headaches, eye pain, nausea, brain fog, heat sensitivity, irritable bowel, peeing problems, numbness, dizziness, anxiety, speech problems, unconsciousness and triggers. And I don't know what more!!

The Invisible Blessing Behind the Pain (Part 11)

By Writer Gargi Sanyal from India

> *"When we lose one blessing,*
> *another is often most unexpectedly given in its place."* ~C.S. Lewis

It took almost 6 months for Gargi to decide to speak to Tonmoy, her husband about her incurable disease. What a terrible dilemma she was undergoing! On one hand was her logical analytical mind: constantly stopping her from disclosing her medical condition with fear of getting misunderstood and mistreated like in her past and again being traumatized and distressed. Though, he had her same emotional never changing mind, seeking for her only love, her only need today.

The one and only who can heal her broken heart, raw wounds, whom she doesn't know why she still loves and wouldn't be able to replace ever! Irrespective of all her fears, every setback, lifelong disrespect, the uncountable broken promises, unbreakable distrust, unhealed hurts, dried up tears, caused by mostly him, her heart even today wants to share everything with him once again.

She feels that if once he embraces her with his hands and hugs her tightly just like that on their wedding night she could at least once more rest her head on his wide shoulders and cry like a baby and open up, her bruised soul would become soothed and relieved from her daily painful unbearable troublesome support less life a little!! The Doctor has repeatedly advised her from the day she was diagnosed with fibromyalgia and chronic fatigue syndrome, an invisible disease, that she needs someone to truly understand her, to love, care for her during her pain, help her heal, share her thoughts and get released from the fear and trauma and stress firstly.

Then only with the help of medicine, good lifestyle like proper diet exercise, stress free happy living, yoga, meditation, relaxation therapies, sufficient sleep, being self-aware as well as making her caregiver aware about leading and living life with this rare complicated fluctuating, of around 200+ symptoms with sudden triggers is truly possible for years. Most of the world are unaware, so also being patient, she should make others aware too. But without that love, no matter how much she tries intensely, ultimately, there's no use as it's the same to say, 'The Countdown Begins!"

She tried to resist her doctor's opinion out of fear but found how true he was when he found her health's deteriorating condition irrespective of being under treatment, as now it was getting reflected on reports too. The other organs had now started getting affected also. Being a mother how can she remain quiet even now. Two little daughters maybe at risk any day if something happens to her. Also, she felt physically and mentally like she was losing all her strengths.

Incidentally she doesn't know why, Tonmoy was also trying to get into touch with Gargi and his two little daughters since a couple of months back directly and indirectly. Sometimes standing in front of the children's school gate suddenly with some gifts to meet them without any occasion, sometimes calling his daughters over the phone suddenly without any purpose just to talk and know how they were doing, or do they need anything, he may try to help if he can, also asking how was their Mamma, wanting to know whether they were still angry upon him? Which he never did since they were separated, and the legal cases were on!

All of us know:

We are here on Earth for a purpose-

for that purpose, to be served by us we are given life,

and how that life is to be led.

God has a plan,

which nobody knows...

Neither Gargi nor Tonmoy knew what had happened to them suddenly!! Maybe they have understood each other, felt their love for each other in their absence, could he realize their own follies, have forgiven each other, maybe not! Maybe they both couldn't bear any more to see the pain in the hearts of their innocent children of being deprived of parents who love together, maybe not! Whatever maybe the reason, it was very clear that they both wanted to reunite or at least speak once to each other before everything was over forever after so many days. And there lied "The Great His Plan!"

Gargi called up Tonmoy at once without losing time. In a trembling voice she started "I, I want to meet you! Have something important. Will you..."

"Yes! Yes of course, why not!!" quickly answered Tonmoy before she could have finished, as if he was waiting for her call a long time ago!

The Invisible Blessing Behind the Pain (Part III)

By Writer Gargi Sanyal from India

"When you focus on being a blessing, God makes sure that you are always blessed in abundance." ~Joel Osteen

This evening! The meeting was scheduled by Tonmoy without delay. This time too, the same place where they met for the last time, 2-yrs back before their separation to speak about it. But now the purpose only the Almighty knows! Sometimes in life it happens, when we just can't understand what to do, but we need to have faith in Him and keep sailing with the winds.

This was exactly the thing happening with Gargi and maybe also with Tonmoy and their two little children. None of them knew the outcome of the meeting, even the topic of discussion wasn't very clear to themselves. Moreover, both were bearing a fearful mind of being misunderstood and losing each other yet again but still both were going to meet their love with a hopeless hope. If something good happens, some miracles, some blessings to be bestowed upon their family of four. They all would be relieved from this undesirable, agony of separation! Maybe still some thin but untorn string of love has remained between both Tonmoy's and Gargi's hearts, which nobody in this world, only the Great-Omnipresent could deny or tear!! Maybe due to that eternal bonding, both today again, are rushing out to meet one another as if it's their first date, also dressing up themselves as if gone back to their teens.

Finally, the clock struck six. The table was pre-booked, Tonmoy was waiting beforehand with a single red rose bud just like in their early days. Gargi entered in her beautiful red gown with her same old shy look through her ever-attractive eyes and a soft smile. Seeing her Tonmoy stood up quickly to greet her and gave his hand to hold, as if Man-and-Wife. After so long by Instinct or by love nobody knows why, Gargi too accepted his hand and walked forward holding his. For some time, both have forgotten their present reality, and had went back a decade of years. The present was here.

Tring-Tring! Gargi's mobile rang suddenly: "Have you reached safely, Meme? Did you find Papa?" -Tinnu called and asked worriedly. "Yes, I am ok, I have met Papa, please don't worry, I'm taking care of myself. You and Binnu, please take care of yourselves, I will be back soon." Gargi hung up the phone. Their dream was over now, it was here. Both then sat face to face in between the harsh reality silently for almost 15 minutes. Then Tonmoy broke the silence stating "You look pretty! Ah, but a little sickly and skinny. Is everything ok? Are you okay, Gargi?" Listening to this she couldn't say a word, only felt a bit emotional and her vision got blurred! She wasn't being able to hold back her tears. He continued "I am truly sorry, I didn't do right to you, and to Tinnu-Binnu.

Will you please forgive and give me another chance to build my family, Gargi? I don't know for what you have called me here today, but I truly wanted to speak to you for a long time! Please come back, I love you, I can't live without you all any longer." While saying Tonmoy didn't notice that Gargi was getting more and more emotional and she was unable to express herself when suddenly she fell and was unconscious. He was shocked to find her like that! Tonmoy immediately took her to the hospital and she was admitted to the emergency. Soon, he called his daughters there.

Finally, he came to know that his wife was dying with fibromyalgia, an incurable invisible disease and chronic fatigue syndrome! Moreover, the cause was the trauma of the emotional and physical absence of her only love, his care and proper understanding, throughout her life which had led her to this approaching death today. And if, and only if that love, care-and-understanding could be present in her life again, then she might survive for many years, along with some support of medicines and a better lifestyle. It was like a nightmare to him. He could never imagine even in his wildest dreams that his absence, his misunderstanding could lead his love to death!

Someone's unawareness can cost one's life! How pathetic it is even to imagine!

He couldn't hold his emotions anymore. He broke down into tears and started sobbing hopelessly while holding his wife tightly to his chest, feeling that she was no more. "I wouldn't let you go this way, Gargi! I will be aware always, will love you, make sure you feel understood to my fullest and make you live for years, and show the world the power of love. I promise! I swear dear! Please-please open your eyes, come back my love!" All-of-a-sudden with the Lord's grace, a faint voice knocked his ears "Please don't cry dear! I am here with you. Just open your eyes and see: Maybe it's not just the invisible disease that I have got, but it's the invisible blessings behind my pain which I have received today, my love! For whatever happens, it happens for some good, and it's my belief, that if it's not the end, then the best is yet to come!"

My Intense Wrangles

By Writer Deborah Denise Lafeber Macias Texas, USA

"To live is to suffer, to survive is to find some meaning in the suffering."
~Friedrich Nietzsche

While my days start out like everyone else's by waking up in the early morning hours, I am dealing with my eyes burning and hurting because they are still so very sleepy. It's as if my body is also still very tired, like a nagging major fatigued tired feeling, as though I just never did rest and have had around six hours of sleep at least. So many nights it's way less and some nights more, it all depends on my mood and my difficult body, I guess. I literally lay there for a long while stretching and opening my eyes and blinking repeatedly thinking, Ugh I really hate mornings and having to wake up because of my eye pains and my achingly stiff joints, muscles, ligaments, and tendons. It really hurts so much to even get out of bed, stand and walk.

Oh my goodness gracious I feel like I'm eighty years old already, because I have to literally force my mind and body every morning to function so I can just get up out of bed and go to the restroom, since that is obviously a must with nature ha-ha... It just really doesn't matter how much I try to rest and sleep because I still must struggle with being so very tired and constantly yawning all day long. It makes me wonder what I can change or do different to better myself and my everyday life. Oh man that just opened up a whole lotta mess for me, and of course it just depressed me more because I just don't have the energy to do much of anything else on top of what I already do as a single Momma, and as life in general gets in my way.

You know what is so very sad to me and really depressing is that I know that I am supposed to immediately thank our precious dear Lord God for even waking me up again and giving me another new day... I sadly am not thinking of being grateful to God at the very moment when I wake up every morning, mostly because I feel so very miserable: nauseous, dizzy, sick feeling, and I usually wake up with a major headache of some sort like a tension, cluster, or stress headache, or just an annoying horrible migraine. I'm still just so very tired that I feel hopeless and miserable because I've been dealing with this for like fifteen years or more. But hey, don't get me wrong here, because I am so very grateful to Jesus Christ for everything in my life, even though I don't always have the best perspective. Although my life is hard, I eventually realize that God is always working things out for my good, in His time of course.

I am often wondering why I must suffer with literally everything in my life, especially my mental and physical health, along with other hard things in my life, but then I think, "Who am I to question God?"

I just have to thank Him for being there with me and holding me up, carrying me most of the time, because I feel in my heart that God is truly the only one that sincerely loves and cares for me, and is the only one that will never hurt me or disappoint me... I say all of that about our Lord because I believe that He is the only one that allows me to really deal with all the mental and physical illnesses. Illnesses that are invisible to most people prevent them from having a heart of understanding, compassion, empathy, or sympathy for people in the same situation as me.

It's a huge struggle and very lonely to be suffering in this way when others don't understand. It would feel a little easier if I visibly looked like something was wrong with me - like if I'd been injured or broke a bone. Honestly though, even when I was visibly suffering, it appeared that people were uncaring even then. I get looks daily when I park in the handicap spaces with my placard. When I get out of the car, I can see that they're wondering what's wrong with me. They don't see the things that I feel inside, or how difficult it is to walk after I've been grocery shopping. Everything I do just causes so much pain and tires me out so easily.

I know that through everything that I am currently suffering, and all that I have already been through, it has shown me that I am a survivor - an overcomer and obviously a persistent fighter. I guess I always have been, but I also have literally given up a few times and hit the very lowest rock bottom. I came to realize the hard way that I had to get back up and fight through all my struggles, even though I must suffer my way out of all the anguish I experience in this life.

I've been told more than once from different people that God obviously still has me here for a reason and He must have huge plans for my future and a better life... So, the main way I deal with all my struggles is in spending alone time with God in prayer daily.

Swollen Glands Gone - Really?

By Author Susan Parker Rosen from Maryland, USA

"All that man needs for health and healing has been provided by God in nature, the challenge of science is to find it." ~**Paracelsus**

When I contracted ME/CFS not much was known about it at all. They called it the Epstein-Barr Virus. You feel as if you are suffering from Monecious but compared to Monecious this virus never goes away. I was approximately 35 or 36 years old when struck down in an office environment, as I described in one of my other stories. I'm 69 at the time of this writing. In 1991 I was involved in a horrible accident and was thrown from the vehicle as we were sideswiped by speeders. Since that accident, which thank god I survived with my two legs (yes, they were going to amputate the left one! Whew am I lucky!). Sitting in an office environment was not something I could do any longer, so I became a sales agent for a vacation company in Ocean City MD. One day a gal that was selling a product for losing weight, figured I try it and purchased some. Well, my first experience was amazing, a miracle occurred!

After just one pill from the supplement that was from a company that I will not mention at this time, there was a huge difference in my health. My horrid, daily, painful, sore, swollen glands were gone! For the first time since that fateful day in the mid-eighties when I became ill with ME/CFS. The next day, of course I took another one, again, my swollen glands are gone. Now at that time it wasn't as if I could discuss it with my doctor. They didn't believe in ME/CFS, shoot neither did they diagnosis Fibromyalgia. But that's for another book. I didn't have a friend with the same disorders back then, that I could talk to about the symptoms. I was alone in this in 2001, without Facebook, without a support system.

So, you are probably wondering if I found this miracle why aren't I sharing the name of the company nor the product? Well, I'm not sure if the company is still around these days, but they soon removed an herb that the FDA deemed unsafe. How did I know it? Simple, when the new stuff the company sold without the herb it didn't work for me anymore. Anxious to find out what was missing from my miracle supplement... I compared bottles. Guess what? The missing herb was ephedra, also known as ephedrine.

Surprised? Imagine how I felt, but it was approximately 2001 when I found relief. 20 years of daily sore glands that felt as if they were as large as a football players neck. They would pop up under my arms, my boobs and my neck. The horrid dragging tired feeling started to lift!

I was no longer affected by CFS/ME. Anytime I felt it come back on, I simply took a small amount by pill. Soon I didn't need to take it at all. Is it a cure? Who knows! All I can say is that it helped me. But please don't do things the way I did.

I had no one to bounce things off back then. Ask your doctor! Seriously. I needed to work for a living and at that time didn't know the dangers of Ephedrine. It's very important that if you use this herb, please ask your doctor about the side-affects. If you have heart issues you don't want to go near it. And there are many side-affects that you need to read about. But if you are told by a medical professional you can take it, try small doses at first as it is a stimulant. You may feel at first as if you drank a ton of very strong coffee. If you are given a green light by a physician then take it easy, seriously. And stay hydrated. Since I found this herb in approximately 2001, I no longer take it. Over time, the symptoms of CFS/ME have disappeared unless I get incredibly stressed. At the time of this writing the drug is legal in the United States.

Ephedra is a medicinal preparation from the plant Ephedra sinica. [1] Several additional species belonging to the genus Ephedra have traditionally been used for a variety of medicinal purposes, and are a possible candidate for the Soma plant of Indo-Iranian religion.[2] It has been used in traditional Chinese medicine for more than 2,000 years.[3][4] Native Americans and Mormon pioneers drank a tea brewed from other Ephedra species, called "Mormon tea" and "Indian tea.".

Wikipedia contributors. (2019, September 25). Ephedra. In Wikipedia, The Free Encyclopedia. Retrieved 17:57, November 1, 2019, from https://en.wikipedia.org/w/index.php?title= Ephedra&oldid=917760882

According to WebMD:

https://www.webmd.com/vitamins/ai/ingredientmono-847/ephedra

How does it work? Ephedra contains a chemical called ephedrine. Ephedrine stimulates the heart, the lungs, and the nervous system.

Post Exertional Malaise

By Author Robin Dix from Maine, USA

You might be asking yourself what on earth is post-exertional malaise? (PEM) Not everyone experiences this, but for those of us who do, it's debilitating. I talked a bit about it in my previous story.

The medical definition of malaise, according to Merriam-Webster, is defined as "an indefinite feeling of debility or lack of health often indicative of or accompanying the onset of an illness."

"Post-exertional means" occurring after exercise or any other type of exertion.

Like all other symptoms we deal with in CFS, this also can vary in intensity and severity. Maybe you worked out too long at the gym or did too much walking on a trip. Maybe you did too much on a day that you felt better, like cleaning your home. For me and many others, it hits when I've walked around a store for 20-30 minutes, or when I take a shower. It takes me several hours, and sometimes days, to feel like myself again.

PEM is not just physical; it also can be mental. If you have a job that requires a lot of thinking or reading for a long period of time, it can become mentally exhausting. I seem to have issues with both. Of course, if I'm physically exhausted, then I also will be at a disadvantage mentally and emotionally.

PEM causes a massive energy crash. It's like hitting a wall and there's no mistaking it when it happens. We are talking about extreme exhaustion, and a potential increase in pain and other symptoms. It is most severe in those of us who not only have CFS, but also fibromyalgia. Suffering with this is one reason I get so frustrated with people who tell me I should exercise more.

Recently, I was at a major department store for well over an hour, walking to the women's department on the opposite side of the huge store, and then searching for the right dress to wear to my son's wedding the next month. I knew I was in trouble when I started limping while leaving the store. I then went straight to the hairdresser for a trim. I was no good for the rest of that day, and for several days after due to PEM. What should have been a fun morning turned into a few horrible days with my CFS.

When I attended my son's wedding, it was a 45-minute car ride each way, 2 plus hours at the reception. Unfortunately, I had to leave before the cake cutting and missed out on most of the fun. I considered it a major victory that I made it! Of course, then I was in bed exhausted for the next several days. I wouldn't have missed that day for anything.

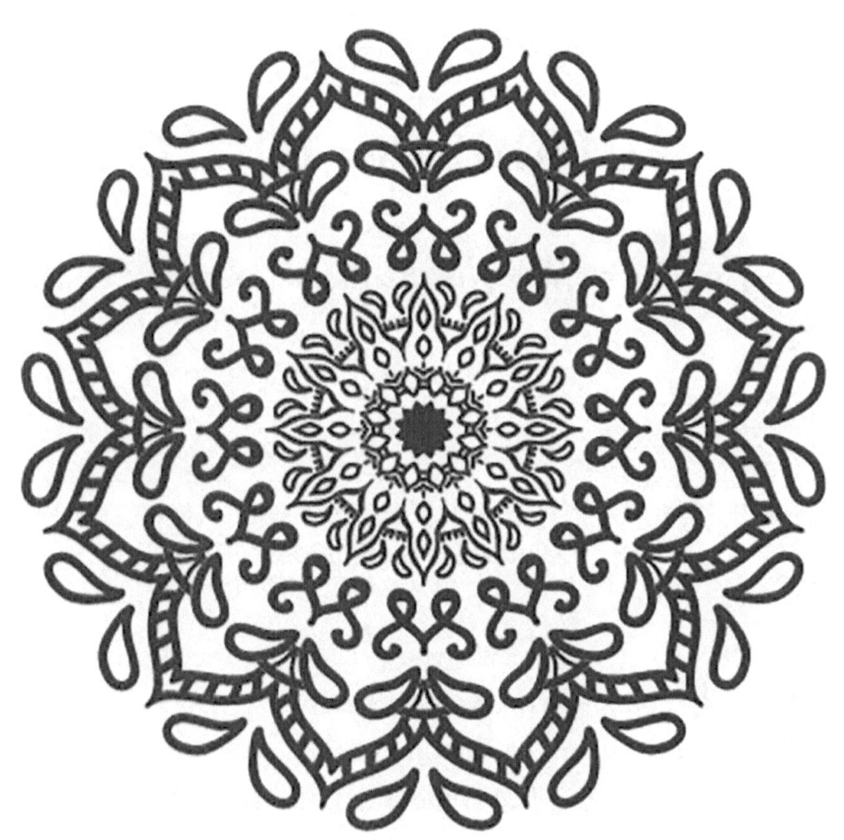

Supposed to Be's

By Writer Kari Ainslie from Ontario, Canada

"Life is supposed to be a series of peaks and valleys. The secret is to keep the valleys from becoming Grand Canyons." **~Bernard Williams**

Do you ever feel like you're taking two steps forward and five thousand steps backward every day? Do you feel like every day is an endless mundane circle, the same activities repeatedly? You lay in bed at the end of the day with the clock passing by the minutes, realizing that it is not simply showing you how to count to fifty-nine. Fifty-nine minutes and then just another thing that repeats again.

Yet, it is also counting by the minutes in life, maybe zooming by, maybe ticking by. You know how they say a "watched pot never boils?" Is it not like that with time? A watched clock never ticks. Tick. Then slowly and eventually, tock. Maybe you look at the forward steps that others are taking announcement about an engagement, a marriage, an expectation of a baby, a job promotion and a raise. Suddenly the minutes fly out the window. Where are all my minutes going? Stop! Hold on! Wait up! There was so much more I wanted to do at this point in my life.

Maybe you look at the backward steps that others are taking: a breakup that is quietly announced, a miscarriage that is grieved, not getting into the school of choice and having to create a new plan, still waiting to meet the right one. Maybe my minutes are just fine. Slow down! Wait! I don't want to waste my minutes waiting for something else, something different. I have the here, and I have the now. Like the glass half empty or half full, I have the choice of how to see these minutes.

Isn't that the most difficult? The idea of it's not supposed to be, or it should be like this feeling. I am sure we all have that. How many times have I pondered: What would my life be like without chronic illness? What decisions would I make? What would I be doing? Where would I be? It's just this imaginary life that is too big to even fathom. Let's take my career projectory as an example.

Maybe I would have stayed in my employment as a Kindergarten teacher. Perhaps I'd still be there full-time and loving it, working hard at lesson content, classroom arrangement (one of my favorites), and experiencing the simple joy of being around children. Or maybe, another reason other than health concerns would have me searching for a new job. Maybe, like in a past employment, I would become restless. There's a possibility that I'd want more things, or perhaps I'd want less. If I apply this principal to everything, I think I am missing out on because of my chronic illness, my life becomes a whole lot of maybes.

So, there is a mourning, a grieving of what is no longer. Sometimes that glass is half empty and I am not too happy about it. Sometimes I feel unaccomplished. A day that has gone by consisting of using all my energy spoons just to do the boring tasks nobody really likes. The restless side of me wants to do more, be more, experience more, dive into more, create more, love more, see more people, see more of life. It occurs sometimes in the night, when I am lying down in the dark, that I'm apt think of all the wonderful things I could be doing. Yet the glass is half empty because my lack of energy has not measured up to all my big plans.

Yet, I allow myself to feel it. I stay there for a while and I mourn. My counselor once described it as a time illustration: "Set a timer," she said. After a while, move on. Sometimes the glass is half full. I speak to myself that I am worthy, important, valued, and loved. I think of one good thing, one thing to be thankful for in this day. I'm proud of myself for being brave and strong, for getting through another hard day of symptoms. I think of all the little things I have time for that working people don't. I think of all the hobbies I've gained. I think of all the other people struggling with illness that I've been able to help. I think of my own story. We all have a story. We all have our it was "supposed to be's."

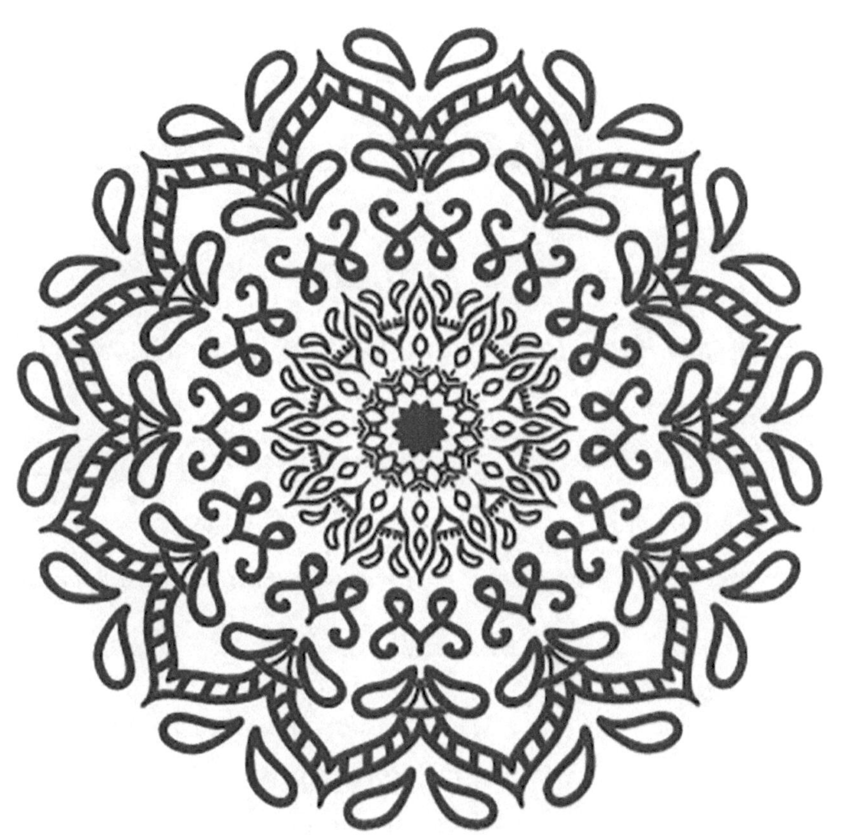

The Window

By Writer

Asha Ryan from Ramsbottom, Lancashire. UK.

"Rivers know this: there is no hurry. We shall get there some day."
~A. A. Milne.

It's week 3 day 3 of a ME/CFS flare up and I have had to 'radically reduce my activity,' as my consultant would advise, in the hope that I can escape a relapse or significantly decrease the intensity and duration of the flare up. So far, my day has consisted of spending the morning in bed and the afternoon lying on the sofa under a duvet.

We have two sofas in our living room. During a flare up where I am predominantly housebound, I alternate between the two sofas. One I use in the morning to do things like read my bible, deal with paperwork, text friends or catch up on emails. A 'doing' sofa if you will. The other one is alongside the window. I use this mainly for watching TV as I can stretch out, on my back, along the sofa, feet up and watch the TV and rest my head on the arm of the sofa if need be. A relaxing TV sofa.

The interesting and sometimes upsetting thing about this 'window' sofa is that I can see and hear what is going on outside. A bit like a fly on the wall. At the end of our road is a school and either side of 9am and 3pm the little cobbled street becomes a hub of activity: parents parked up either waiting in their cars or getting out or getting back in again, other parents walking to and from school with school kids in tow, or just babies and toddlers post drop off. I hear all sorts, the kids shouting in excitement, a mum playing peekaboo trying to entertain the babies while they wait, the dull but rhythmic thud of music as stereos help pass the time until kids can be dropped or collected from school.

This is the worst time of the day to be on the window sofa, but often I am here in the afternoon watching TV or trying to, depending on how bad my burning eyes are or how bad my headache is. I often pull one curtain slightly to protect my eyes from the bright daylight but also, I realize, because I feel quite ashamed and embarrassed, that I am just sitting there.

Once I have dropped my daughter off at school I come home and bounce between these two sofas and my bed all day until it is time to go and pick her up. Sometimes I can't manage to take her to school or pick her up and someone steps in for me, it is at these times that I feel my illness most keenly. Unfortunately for me, witnessing this hustle and bustle creates a complete sensory overload and all my sensitivities seem to come into play.

The kids crying is suddenly too shrill, the adults talking is too loud, the banging of the car doors make me jump and all I want to do is open the front door and ask them to please keep the noise down.

Despite how I feel, I try to remember that these people are oblivious to me being there and my condition. It is not their fault and I try to cultivate some compassion for these people, because they are just living their lives and going about their business.

I am not a bitter person, usually I am friendly, joyful and celebrating of people and life, but this illness at times robs me of any joy. I even hear myself silently cursing the lady next door whose laugh is 'too' loud. How dare she be happy while I convalesce on the sofa for the third week running, struggling to get myself up to go to the toilet or to make that cup of tea. That feeling, incidentally, is often followed by a prayer to God asking for forgiveness for my resentment, jealousy and coveting of her joy.

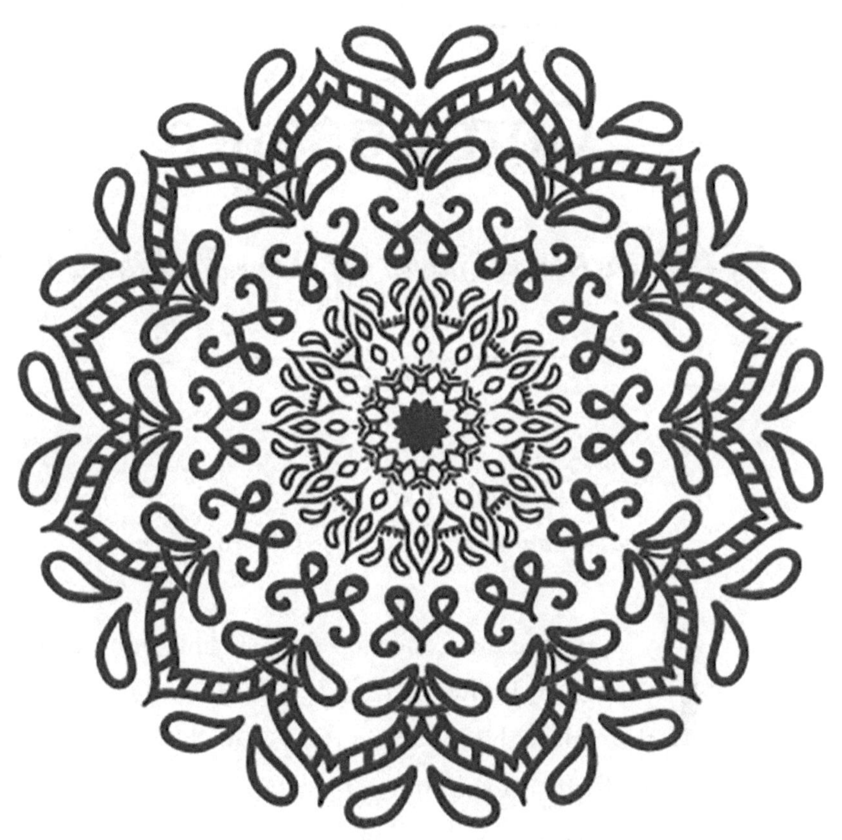

Compassion

By Author Donna Short RN from Michigan, USA

"The emotion that can break your heart is sometimes the very one that heals it..." ~**Nicholas Sparks**

My eyes open to another day. Thank you, God. Even though I know each day will be tough and pushed through with everything I physically have, I am grateful. I to focus on the things I can do. It has taken a while to learn this and to change my thinking to the positive. It's like crafting a fine art, learning to play a Cello, or learning a new language. Every day before I get out of bed, I always ask myself, I wonder what today will bring? It's kind of like a game. What is ME/CFS going to bring my way today. I am a warrior, bring it on! I fight through it all and push myself to my maximum physical ability without going into a flare. Like walking a tightrope, always on that fine line.

I often push to far, but I can't help it, my pride is on the line; my ego, expectations, not wanting to fail at anything, competitiveness, my health, socialization, family, friends. Pretty much everything! When I push, I pay. The exhaustion is overwhelming! It grabs ahold of me and just drains my energy from head to toe. I feel like I weigh a ton, I can't keep my eyes open, and my muscles are burning and weak. I feel as though I am doing a full body workout on the last set and last rep, the burning and extreme weakness always wins. Exhaustion always puts me to bed, sometimes too weak to even text someone or play a game on my phone. I have no choice but to wave my white flag and surrender to it and that's okay.

I must listen to my body, no matter what my brain wants to do. My brain says; "Let's go to the gym, or do some stuff around the house, work in the yard, hang out with friends, go shopping, have my hair or nails done." My body laughs like it's saying "Ha! That's not going to happen, and neither are basic activities of daily living, like showering!" I have learned my bodies limits. I know that when my arms or legs start to burn and feel like jello that it is time to rest. As much as I hate it, I do it. I know if I don't sleep well at night that I need to take it easy the next day, or if I have an event to attend, I have learned to take it easy the day before to hopefully have energy to even attend the event.

I have a mild/moderate case of ME/CFS. I count that as a blessing, it could be worse! One thing that I have noticed is that people do not understand or comprehend how being around people and socializing is exhausting. First, we must put on our "I feel good mask" when we socialize. No one wants to be around someone that is literally miserable, doesn't smile, winces in pain, can't stay awake and must fake being well. It's draining! We are dealing with extreme exhaustion, pain, and more, so that alone knocks our batteries down to fifty percent. So, add talking, laughing, faking to be normal, I am a great actress of my craft. No one has ever been able to define normal, but normal as in being able to have a career, a family, socialize and not have to force a smile. Balance. Enjoying this journey until we pass over to the next.

The word compassion has recently been laid on my heart, we need so much more compassion in the world today. You don't know what people are going through. There are so many invisible illnesses. I think of the old days when friends, family, and neighbors would help someone when they needed it. Without having to ask or made to feel weak or broken as an individual. It's the small things; bring a meal over, text to see how we are or if we need anything, or just say hello, a grocery run, clean the bathroom, maybe a little housework if they are behind, picking up our meds from the pharmacy, a listening ear, or a smile and a hug. We are not looking for sympathy. Simple, little things that say I am here for you! Compassion.

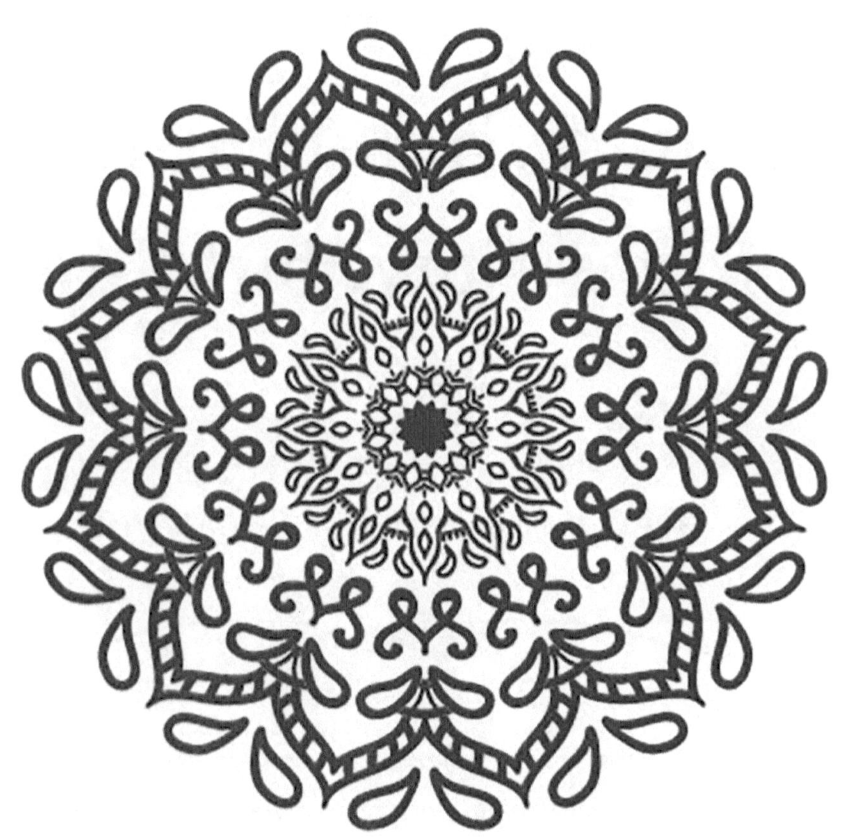

I Can't Stand For Long Right Now, but I Am Not Giving up on Me

By Author Abby Guss from Ohio, USA

"It doesn't matter how high you climb the mountain, it's the view that's beautiful." **~Missi Page Prestwood**

At the age of 40, I was finally diagnosed with Chronic Fatigue Syndrome and advanced Adrenal Fatigue. While it was nice to get a diagnosis, one I knew I already had, there is no cure or recognized protocol to treat someone with a "ghost illness". For at least 12 years, I have noticed a progression of medical symptoms, all of which were disregarded by physicians. I did my part in trying to get help, and now, I am suffering.

This has been a long time coming, but my body finally gave. I ran a 5K, and the week after I couldn't climb the stairs. Then I couldn't even drive, followed by 2 months of being bed ridden. Some days I couldn't walk at all, my legs felt so heavy I physically couldn't move them. It was maddening, and in addition, who I thought was my greatest love left me, too. Where do you go from there?

I am now 42, and while I have a new knowledge base, I am still exhausted, still have trouble maintaining work with my brain fog, and now I cannot stand long. I should be at a prime with healthy bloodwork, yet I cannot stand upright for a long time. I have gone from a go-getter to a wasted decade of my 30s to now being in bed.

Some days I can walk a mile, others I can't walk to the end of the driveway. If I clean too much, I must rest. If I try to exercise, I know the next day I'll be exhausted. If I eat gluten or soy or dairy or dessert or eat out, my body will cause a ruckus.

Some days I try to ignore things and hope they will get better, but it is just to keep my sanity. The other night in choir about did it for me. The director wanted us to stand at the beginning of rehearsal for a classical piece, understandably. I couldn't do it. I am 42, and I couldn't stand. In my brain I kept saying, get up, get up! Yet, I couldn't. I had to constantly keep sitting down and resting. I had to rest for two minutes into a choir rehearsal. That is maddening. I also cannot do work that requires too much standing or walking, and an 8-hour workday seems so foreign to me.

So, with all that exhaustion and limitation, where do I go from here? There doesn't seem to be a solution or help, let alone a cure. I keep trying, I keep falling and failing, yet I keep an eye out some other supplement or breakthrough. I don't know about you, but I am kind of tired of all the seemingly chronic negative aspects of my body. I am tired of what my body can't seem to do. So! I decided to change as best I can in how I look at it.

I am waking up every day with a renewed gratitude that I awoke. Maybe today I won't be able to walk far, maybe today I have a hard time thinking or moving, and maybe today the best I have is to cry it out. I just know I have been living in an emotional prison with an incredibly limited body, and this girl is tired of it. I am choosing to celebrate every victory, no matter how seemingly small, and making the effort to love me again. I will find the plan to revamp my body, one step at a time.

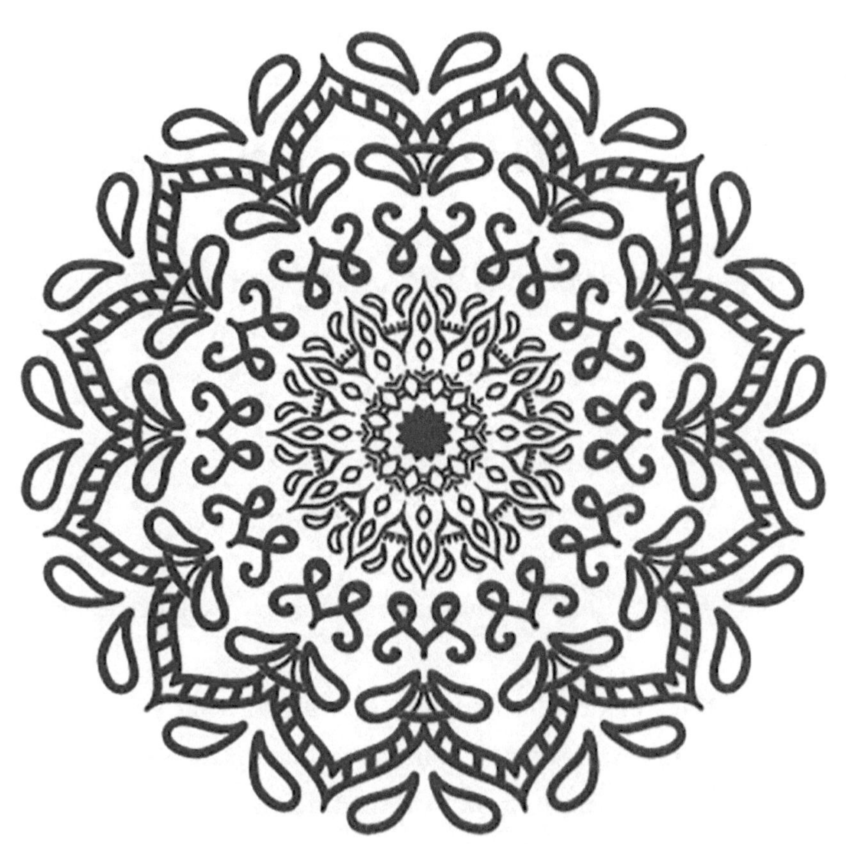

Whine or Wine

By Author Jeanne Getz Pallos from California, USA

"Laugh at yourself and at life. Not in the spirit of derision or whining self-pity, but as a remedy, a miracle drug, one that will ease your pain…Never take yourself too seriously." **~Og Mandino**

"It's anxiety," the urgent care doctor told me as I explained my symptoms. "Go home and take a Xanax and have a glass of wine." As tears streamed down my face, he said, "Well, have wine with Xanax." I cried all the way to my car. How could anyone feel this sick and have nothing wrong? Why couldn't he believe me? My daughter had just been married two months earlier. I'd spent months helping her plan the December 29th destination wedding. Besides the wedding, I hosted Christmas, arranged pet sitting, packed, and left for the wedding two days after Christmas. The days were filled with rehearsals, dinners, and meeting new family members.

Daily I begged God: Please help me not get sick. Help me to get through this.

Now, I sat in front of a doctor who did not believe that I was sick. How could I be? Blood tests always came back normal, so it must be anxiety or depression. I first heard of chronic fatigue syndrome in the 1980s. When I went to a doctor with a list of my symptoms, he told me that I was depressed and the most compulsive/obsessive person he'd ever met. That was the first time I drove home from a doctor's office in tears. My husband and I attended a lecture on this new disease. The speaker explained my symptoms perfectly. "On good days, you are convinced you don't have this disease. You sign up for classes at the junior college; buy paint to paint your house; plan a trip. Then, you crash."

That was me. When I felt good, I convinced myself that I did not have CFS. My motto was: When the sun shines, I make hay. Although CFS was getting some recognition, I discovered that mainstream doctors did not recognize it as a disease. I went from doctor to doctor looking for answers and validation. Eventually, I went into intense therapy. Why did I need this disease? How did it benefit me? Was it in my head? Was it depression? Therapy took me deep into my life issues, and I was determined to recover my health. I learned ways to acknowledge my feelings and establish better relationships. I worked to uncover every possible reason that I needed to be sick. Therapy gave me new methods of dealing with stress and anxiety, but CFS still ran the show. When I over exerted, I paid the price of weeks or months in bed.

Leaving the urgent care that day, I felt alone in my suffering as ever. Why did I bother trying to be understood? This was a private disease. I no longer even told people that I had CFS. I simply said, "I have health limitations." I finally found a doctor who believes me. He says, "I know you are sick. We just don't know what it is. One day, we will." Until that day, I'll try not to whine. My doctor rules out other illnesses when I am in a full blown CFS episode. For now, that is good enough.

Too Many Pillows

By Writer Jennifer Bartholomew from Illinois, USA

"People will never truly understand something until it happens to them."
~Unknown

You will never get it, till you get it. A saying that fell on deaf ears until a few years ago. I'm embarrassed to admit, I was that person who saw someone in an electric scooter or wheelchair that could walk and thought "Why in the world does an able-bodied person use that?" "Aren't those for paralyzed or elderly people?" I was uninformed, judgmental and opinionated. Not because I was cruel or mean spirited, I just didn't know anything about the world of invisible illness.

I tend to believe this is the case for most people who haven't lived with chronic illness, namely ME/CFS. You just don't get it, till you get it. My time is spent being sedentary, usually in my bed. On better days or in better moments I can be on a sofa or sit up for a while. Long gone are the days of gallivanting around like the social butterfly I once was. I traded in my stilettos for slippers and sequin tops for soft jammies. My life is simple these days. Everything I do depends on my ability to function, be it cognitively or physically, most days both are lacking. On the days my brain seems to be firing decently I spend my time writing, communicating with friends and loved ones, and being of service in any way I can.

You'd be surprised what it can do for your mental health to just be available and love someone through what they are going through! I've found many like-minded people online who have become friends, family, and confidants. Amazing people who also fight chronic pain and illnesses, people I would have never had in my life had I never gotten sick. I'm grateful for every moment I've had the chance to interact and get to know them, they are my lifeline to the world!

Then there are the bad days. Those days when my pain is unmanageable, my symptoms have peaked, and I'm too weak to fight. I hide away, tucked into my room, snuggled in bed with as many pillows as I can manage, maybe even too many pillows. Passed out from fatigue or awake with painsomnia, I have to relinquish control and be at the mercy of ME/CFS. I imagine myself cut off from the world, an island at sea, abandoned. Nothing to offer, a burden, a boil on the rear of society. These are some of the emotions and thoughts I struggle with while my body spasms and indescribable pain courses through every inch of me. My skin hurts and prickles at the air, my joints ache and swell, connective tissues inflamed, even my organs hurt.

Then there are the symptoms. There's so many, a list would be impossible. Dr. Karen Klimas an ME researcher and clinician at the University of Miami is quoted as saying "ME/CFS patients experience a level of illness and disability equal to those with end stage AIDS and patients undergoing chemotherapy." We never know when something will happen that changes us, and our life, forever. It happens on a dime, in the blink of an eye, a nanosecond.

What I've learned from how ME/CFS has changed my life, is that people can look like they're just going through their day. Just another face in the crowd. Yet, underneath the smile they may be suffering from things they never share, invisible things. Always practice kindness, always love, and always appreciate every moment you have...even if you must do it from a bed piled high with too many pillows.

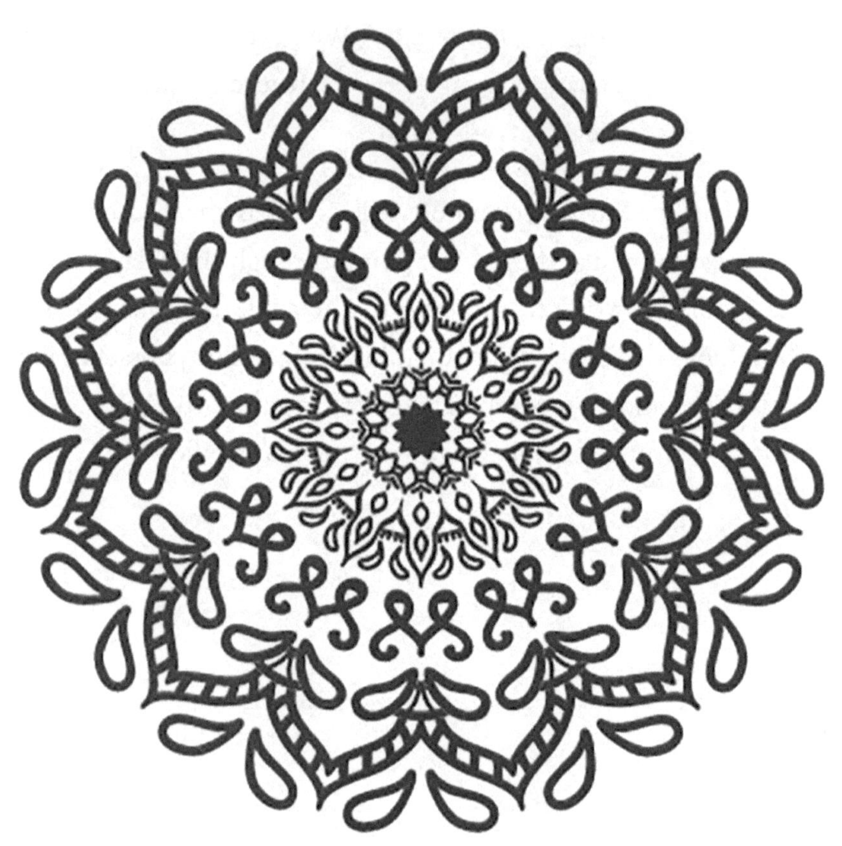

The Challenges of CFS

By Author Robin Dix from Maine, USA

> *"We've documented, as have others, that the level of functional impairment in people who suffer from CFS is comparable to multiple sclerosis, AIDS, end stage renal failure, chronic obstructive pulmonary disease. The disability is equivalent to that of some well-known, very severe medical conditions."*
>
> ~Dr. William Reeves, former CDC Chief of Viral Diseases Branch

There are so many things I still struggle with that ten years ago would not even have been on my radar. When you're healthy there are so many things to take for granted. It's only when you gradually lose the ability to do them that your world begins to shrink. CFS is a tough task master!

I used to keep a very clean home, even when my children were small. The bathrooms were cleaned weekly, I dusted once a week, I was even able to do spring and fall cleaning. I enjoyed cleaning! Now if I dust one room, it wipes me out for hours afterwards. My husband has taken over all the cleaning and I'm so grateful. Otherwise my home would be a disaster. I can do laundry. Even if I'm too tried to take clothes out of the dryer that day, the next day that I feel well enough I just put the dryer on 'wrinkle release' and then fold and put away. I mostly wear comfy dresses, so there's not much folding to do. Whew!

Dressing can be another challenge. When my bursitis in my shoulder flares, my husband must help me as I'm unable to lift one or both arms. It's especially difficult in the winter when I must wear a coat. I just must be mindful of putting in the incapacitated arm first. There are times that it makes me feel like a child, having to have someone help me get dressed and tie my shoes for me. Walking used to be my favorite exercise, taking long walks helped me relax and gave me time to think and pray without distractions.

These days if I walk too much not only do I tire easily, but my right arthritic hip begins to hurt and before you know it, I'm limping. I'm thankful for my medical devices that enable me on days that are incredibly difficult. Recently my husband and I went to the store to pick up a few things when suddenly I started to feel weak and ill. I told my husband to go pay and I'd go out to the car (thank God for handicapped parking), but true to his nature he found me a nearby bench in the store and had me sit while he went to get me an empty cart to help me walk out of the store. Then he went with me to be sure I got there ok and turned on the AC to keep me comfortable before going back in the store to pay.

Keeping up with the activities of daily living (ADL) is so hard! There was a time that I showered and styled my hair AND put on makeup. Now I'm lucky I feel up to taking a shower once a week because I know there will be hours of down time after that. My husband enjoys washing my hair, which is great because it's much less tiring to have him do it than when I do it myself. I do a lot of sponge baths right before I turn in for the night. I keep wipes on hand for when I can't even manage that. I used to embrace all the challenges that came my way, thinking up creative solutions. These days my creativity is sorely challenged by CFS and its comorbidities. Although every day is a struggle, I refuse to give up or give in. I choose to be a warrior!

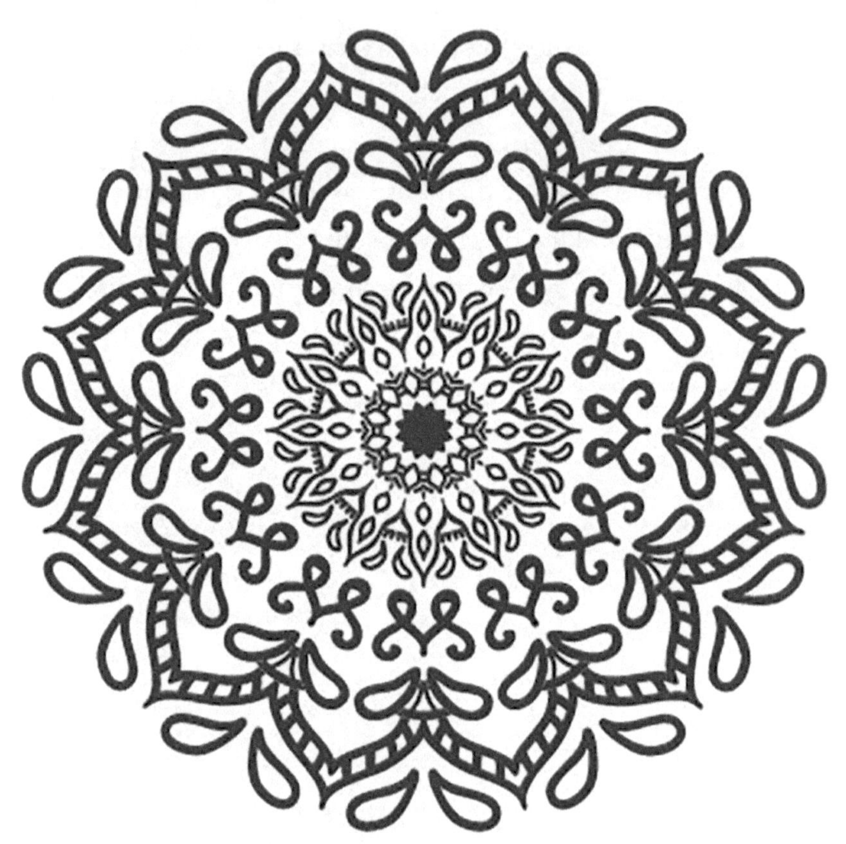

The Invisible Girl

By Kari Ainslie from Ontario, Canada

*"Chronic fatigue syndrome can turn
a life of productive activity into one of dependency and desolation."*
~ Jose Montoya, M.D. Stanford University

"I had been getting better, but then I crashed again. I've been feeling so sick in my bed since Saturday night. The Doctors are saying they don't know, can't find anything wrong. Some doctors make me feel like I am mentally insane. Test after test is normal, so this must all be in my head. It's like unless they got into my body, they won't understand or comprehend. They don't get why I won't just 'snap out of it.'"
~ (My Diary, November 30, 2015)

What's it like having an invisible illness? It's like carrying a giant backpack around that's filled with bricks. It's way too heavy for you, and you know it's too heavy, but no one around you will stop to ask if you'd like some help carrying it, because they can't even see that you are. If you had a giant pile of luggage at an airport, it would be rude for other people not to stop and offer you some kind of assistance: an extra hand, one of those special carts with the wheels, point you towards the elevator. In a life carrying a backpack that no one else can see, you must specifically ask for all the things that you need. It would be nice if you could be met with a "Oh yeah, that looks heavy! Here, let me help you!" Instead, you're often awarded with strange stares. You know their thoughts, even if they don't speak them. If they do, they question you.

It can be a lonely life. Sometimes it's easier to carry that backpack alone. Every few steps, you must stop to take a break. You open the backpack to see if you can let out any of the contents. "It all stays," you say. You pick it up and begin again. Carrying this backpack isn't temporary. Unlike in an airport, you're not sure when you'll reach the destination and be able to place it down. No one can give you a timeline or a treatment, a projected duration. You never know if you'll get better or if you'll get worse. So, you must pick it up again, even though it's the same weight as before, and the break times become more and more frequent. It's taking you so long to do everything with this huge weight upon yourself that nothing much is getting done. The 'to do' list grows, daunting and leaving you with disappointment. There is a mourning, a missing of the normal.

I wrote this poem 'Invisible Girl' before I got ill, but I thought it was a great way to describe the feelings of what it is like to have an invisible illness. It's a feeling where you worry, you're disappearing into the crowd, or not disappearing into any crowd because the 'crowds' that you used to be a part of eventually stop asking why you do not come to certain events. The normalcy of a life of social engagements becomes a life of balancing that backpack, weighing when you can go, and sometimes when you simply cannot. As you're carrying that heavy backpack, each step feels like the weight of it is just too much, too heavy. Yet you must be amazingly strong to keep going.

You say she's just a girl

that you sometimes see around

and you never wonder,

or decide to make a sound,

because she's just another face

disappearing in the crowd,

and she walks through you

and she's never very loud.

She's just another name

that you no longer know.

You never acknowledge her

and you think she doesn't realize so.

She's just another person,

although she once was more;

It's just that now she walks,

instead of being able to soar.

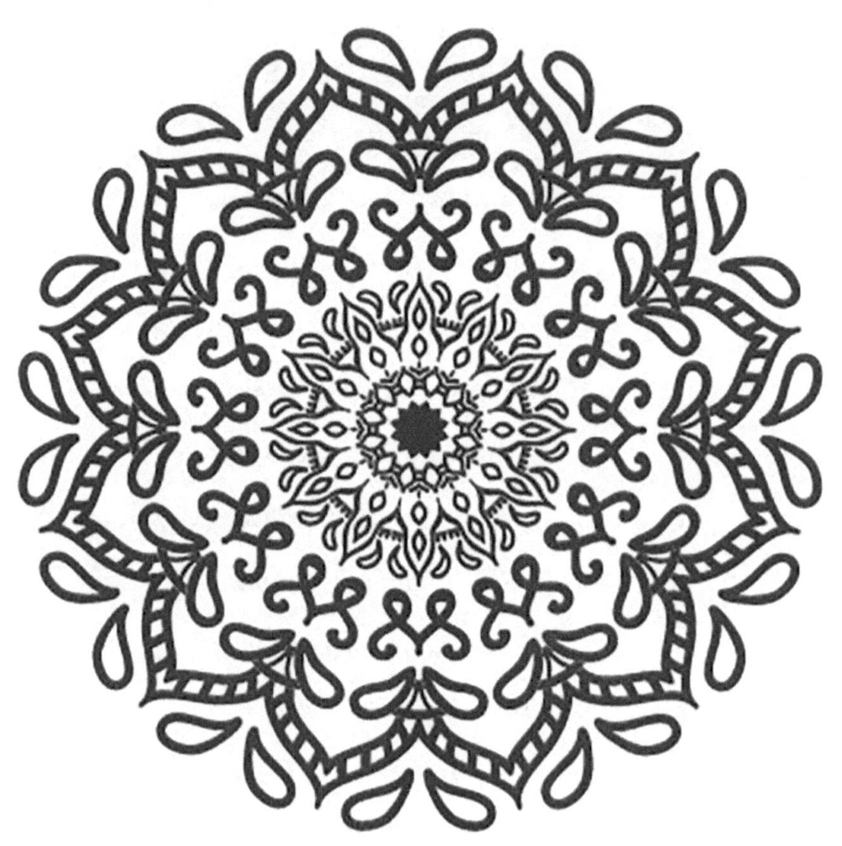

Feeling Better

By Writer Asha Ryan from Ramsbottom, Lancashire, UK

"Yet what we suffer now is nothing compared to the glory he will reveal to us later." ~Romans 8:18 NLT

"Are you feeling better?" seems like a fairly innocent question, but for me, and I imagine many others with a chronic condition, it is actually quite a complicated question. Every time someone asks me if I am feeling better, I hesitate. I hesitate, because although I have managed a week or two of trying my normal routine, post flare up, my health and energy are very much on a moment by moment basis. Some activities I haven't been able to do at all. Yet this is what recovery from a flare up looks like. So, if someone asks me if I am feeling better, I have a dilemma. Do I say yes because I am no longer in a flare up or do I reply honestly with how I'm feeling at the moment?

As it happens, I do tend to reply honestly, but every time I do it, it does make me think. It makes me think about what it means to 'feel better' for a person with CFS like me. I have to think of my energy a bit like a bank account, if I spend some of that energy on one activity then I have less to spend elsewhere. I also need to think about if I can increase my energy in any way. Like an income, can I put any energy back in the bank, by resting or engaging in extremely low level activities.

Sometimes I am pleasantly surprised by how quickly I can recover my energy after an activity, and I guess that is what a 'recovery' period feels like – being able to recover energy at a normal rate or speedier rate than before. At other times though it is not favorable, and an activity can lead to a significant requirement for rest, or a relapse in symptoms and the recovery time is then much longer.

In terms of planning a week's activities, it is a very fine balance of trying to guess how much energy one activity might use and estimate the recovery time, based on when I might comfortably be able to commit to the next activity. As I say though, this kind of planning is easily thrown out if my estimated recovery time is longer than anticipated. That then leads to a domino effect on other activities scheduled for that week, leading me to cancel activities or reschedule tasks for later in the week.

On Monday mornings I facilitate a group called Mindful Mondays. The group aims to help people ease into their week and provide a support network for those, including myself, who don't fit into the normal Monday to Friday working pattern. It's been a bit touch and go the last few weeks as it depends very much on my health as to whether or not I can facilitate the weekly group.

In the lead up to each Monday I tend to keep evaluating my health on a daily basis to see if I think I might be able to do it. If I do run it, I must think about how long it might take me to recover afterwards and tie that recovery in with other activities that I might have committed to that week. Often if I do one thing then I have to cancel another. It's a constant juggling act. What I do know though, is that God is with me every step of the way and that His plan for each and every one of us is far greater than we can ever imagine. Despite the suffering, I like to think we are all serving a purpose, and that can help us feel better.

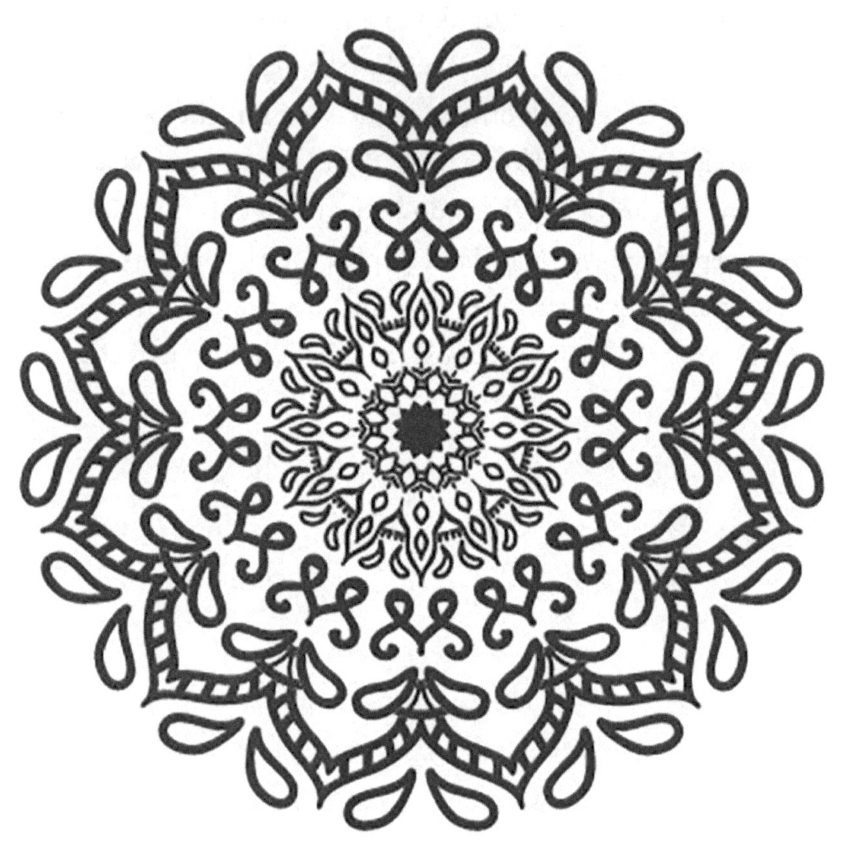

Switch!

By Author Donna Short RN from Michigan, USA

"You wake up every morning to fight the same demons that left you so tired the night before, and that, my love, is bravery." **~Unknown**

In January 2012 I was diagnosed with fibromyalgia and then in 2014 followed a diagnosis of chronic fatigue syndrome. I have knowledge of fibromyalgia learning from patients as a nurse, but ' What the heck is that and what does it mean? In other words, the first thing I want to know is how to get rid of it! I love doing research, I am a very curious person naturally and I need to know how things work and what makes people tick. Physiology, here I come! Wow was I shocked! All I knew was that I went to the doctor with: loss of memory, decreased concentration, a very sore throat, large lymph nodes in my neck, pain from head to toe, headaches almost daily, never feeling refreshed in the morning, and extreme exhaustion after physical exercise or mental stress.

The next thing I know is that I'm learning that CFS is chronic! I'm thinking "are you kidding me?" "Really?" I guess having fibro wasn't enough. I kept reading and learned that fibro and CFS are a lot alike except with CFS you also have the symptoms listed above. Fibro is more pain, CFS is more exhaustion in my case. Finally, after about four years I have been able to tell the difference between a fibro flare compared to a CFS flare. With my CFS I tend to start feeling a sore throat coming on more painful than usual and my muscles become weak, especially my arms, legs, and hands. My jaw gets tired from chewing, and I become grumpy because I am so tired, my cheeks feel fatigued from smiling or laughing, and I can only handle so much stimulation and that's when I usually end up in bed.

I often fall sleep from exhaustion, but I also just lay there resting at times. I will either watch television or think about how much this sucks, and all the things I can't do anymore. I lost my job because I couldn't write anymore, had to give my motorcycle back to the bank because I couldn't ride it nor afford it now, I often need to take breaks between showering, drying off, and getting dressed. I loved to run, nope that's out. I can't keep up with the housework anymore and often need help. I'm pooped by two pm, so that's when my day is usually over and it's time to rest. I think about how lost I feel, and sad. No social life, and a loss of friends, because I'm just not as fun as I used to be.

One day while lying in bed "resting" I decided I had two choices. One, lay around thinking horrible thoughts and making myself feel like a useless burden, or two, try to find things that I enjoyed that I can do. I tried so many things, arts and crafts, and I learned about different religions because I felt so lost. I tried to play the harmonica, but my dogs would have no part of that and would howl so loud I couldn't hear what I was trying to learn to play. I tried crocheting, not only boring but my hands and forearms became fatigued with the repetitive movement. I made candles with essential oils....meh, not really my thing.

Finally, I decided I had to change my thinking from what I can't do to what I can do. I switched my focus and I started thinking positively. It's harder said than done indeed, but I definitely wasn't going to make my situation miserable. I started making sure I got enough sleep and started practicing self-love. If I couldn't sleep, I would watch something educational or listen to an audio book. I started to learn energy conservation, as well as positive thinking, and just randomly smiling because there is always something to be grateful for. The mind is a powerful thing, and I am surely not going to waste mine. I intend to accomplish great things, and that my friends, is bravery.

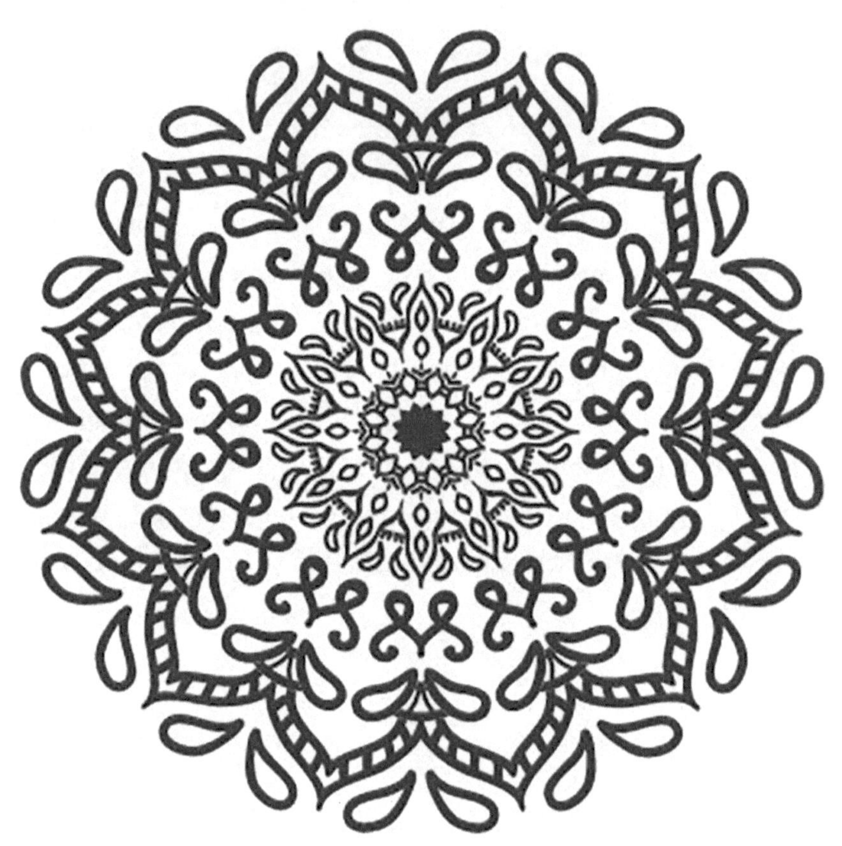

Fail More and Fail Better: I Am the Boss of Me

By Author Abby Guss from Ohio, USA

"Don't worry about failures, worry about the chances you miss when you don't even try." ~Jack Ganfield

A year and a half ago I was officially diagnosed with chronic fatigue syndrome and advanced adrenal fatigue. In addition to being hypoglycemic, having a thyroid issue and debilitating depression and anxiety, I had a diagnosis to what I already knew. I have a chronic metabolic syndrome that strips my body of energy, and medical professionals seem to be grabbing at straws. I was newly single, trying to muster enough energy to get some work done and get through my day as best my body would allow. I took a trip to a state park for a renewed spirit and clarity of mind, well what a fogged brain could do.

I read a book entitled "Fail, fail again, fail better," by Pema Chödrön. She stated, "That it is okay to face the unknown, and what if we become a more complete person during the process?" I thought, I CAN fail again, I do it every day! Sometimes life doesn't give us what we would like, so we are to lean into the uncertainty. Hmmm.... it's kind of difficult to focus on positivity when your body is giving out on you leading to depression, anxiety and panic attacks. I was going to give it a better try. I had to, because I just didn't have anything left in the fight. Maybe "the fight" was the problem.

I decided to make a solid commitment to flip my thought process. Instead of what I couldn't do, why not focus on what I could? I was able to walk a mile the other day, and while my time didn't improve, I thought you are out here! Your time didn't get worse it was the same, you were healthy enough to go, now drink your water and try again tomorrow!

In that mile I had accomplished a lot. I got off the couch, I did some activity, I walked more, tried more, and most importantly, I didn't go down the rabbit hole of what I couldn't or didn't do. My body went as far as it could, and I was respecting it.

I knew if my body was to be so acutely respected, I had to get completely organized. It is easy to let a lot go during a good round of exhaustion and depression. I was committing to a new long-term process. Solidly committing to wellness no matter what really changed the game for me.

Food. Food is a huge component, and while I had long ago switched to organic and grass-fed or wild caught everything, I hadn't been consistent with my eating schedule. I use a food app to keep me honest.

Water. There was a new hydration schedule. I live in a cold area of the country, so it is easy to become dehydrated. Filtered water and organic juicing were to be better organized.

Sleep. I made myself get ready earlier for bed, changed around my bedroom to make it a happier place, and made my bed every day. I knew I wouldn't want to mess up a made bed as much, and if I needed rest, it was okay!

Acupuncture. This is a therapy that costs a car payment a month but is crucial for my anxiety and wellbeing.

Proper supplementation scheduling. I found that physician grade supplements were far ahead of what was available in stores.

While this seems like a full-time job to keep my body healthy, it's a must for my wellness. I am committed to what works best for me, regardless of what anyone thinks or says. You got this!

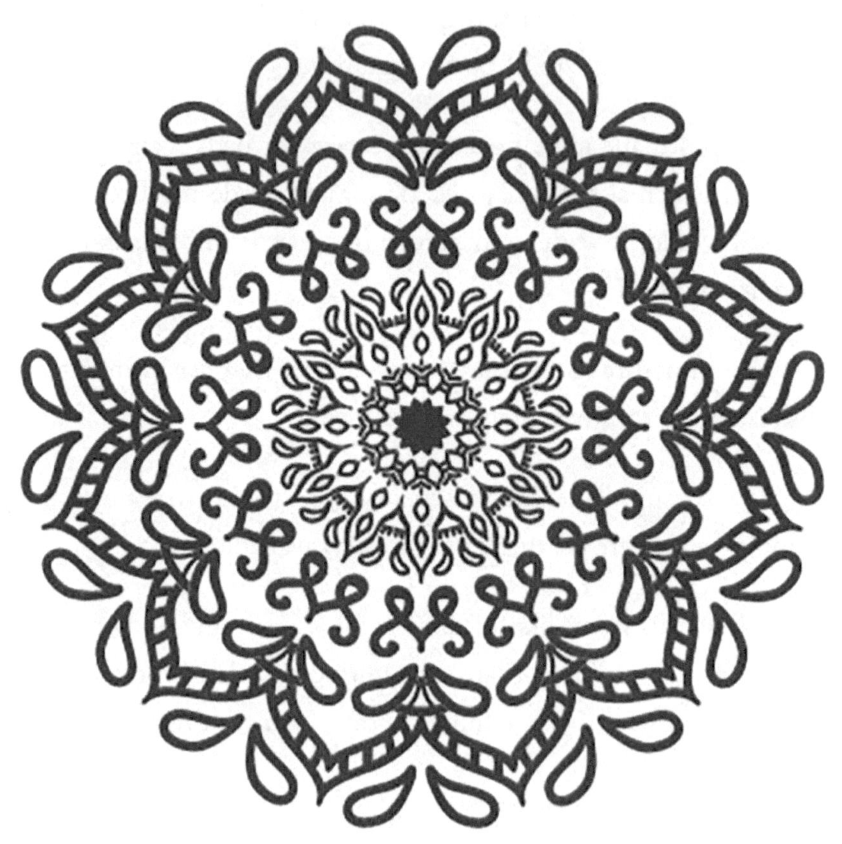

The Name Game

By Author Jeanne Getz Pallos from California, USA

> *"A rose by any other name would smell as sweet..."*
> **~William Shakespeare**

The title of the newspaper article caught my attention: chronic fatigue syndrome has a new name, possibly a new test. I had been searching for answers to my non-disease since the 1980s. This article had some new insights. The first paragraph told me what I already knew—chronic fatigue syndrome was a hated name. Nor was it considered a real disease. Now, the independent Institute of Medicine was giving CFS a new name: SEID (Systemic Exertion Intolerance Disease) that reflected the major symptom—exertion wipes us out. Dr. Ellen Wright Clayton assured a panel of experts that we have a real disease and our symptoms aren't imagined. We deserve real care. Yet, according to the article, less than a third of medical schools teach about the disease.

After I finished reading, my mind drifted back over the years. I went from doctor to doctor searching for a reason that I was more tired than most people. Tired, in this case, is a very weak word. Most days, I felt like I was wearing heavy construction boots and walking through wet cement. Other days, I imagined myself loaded with heavy backpacks filled to the brim and forced to climb a mountain. I had two young children and a husband establishing a dental practice. Our son was a two-year-old toddler and our daughter a three-month-old infant when my husband decided to leave a secure job and go to dental school. My health had been fragile from the beginning of our marriage, but I was still able to teach school. Now that we had children, my health would not permit me to work.

Without family or friends to help, I dragged through the days. At night, I nursed my daughter and resented that she kept me from sleeping. Long days and sleepless nights wore down my body and soul. Why could other young mothers care for their children, plus work outside the home? One woman in my husband's class gave birth over the Christmas break and was back in school full time when classes resumed in January. I couldn't begin to imagine having that kind of capacity. My health never recovered once my husband finished school and started his practice. Yet, I tried to be like every other mother.

I drove carpool, threw birthday parties, put our kids in soccer, swimming, gymnastics, and diving. One year, we hosted an exchange student. Another year, I was the soccer team mom. On the days I couldn't get out of bed, friends picked up the kids and drove carpool for me. Doctors could find nothing wrong. Every test came back normal. I prayed for a diagnosis. How could I feel this sick and have nothing wrong? Outwardly, I looked fine. Inwardly, I wondered if I'd live to raise my kids. Yes, it was that bad. Reading the article gave me a sense of validation. Yes, I really was sick. My suffering was real. A new name doesn't change anything. There is no cure.

Most doctors still don't believe CFS exists. According to their training, tests never lie. My doctors treat different aspects of the disease when I have a flare-up. It's like swatting at flies. What caused this latest collapse? How do I get back on my feet? Will it last days, weeks, or months? I've been dealing with this disease for over thirty years. For most of those years, it had no name. I felt isolated, alone, and misunderstood. Now, we have a new name and a few people who believe in us. Chronic fatigue syndrome by any other name is just as miserable and misunderstood.

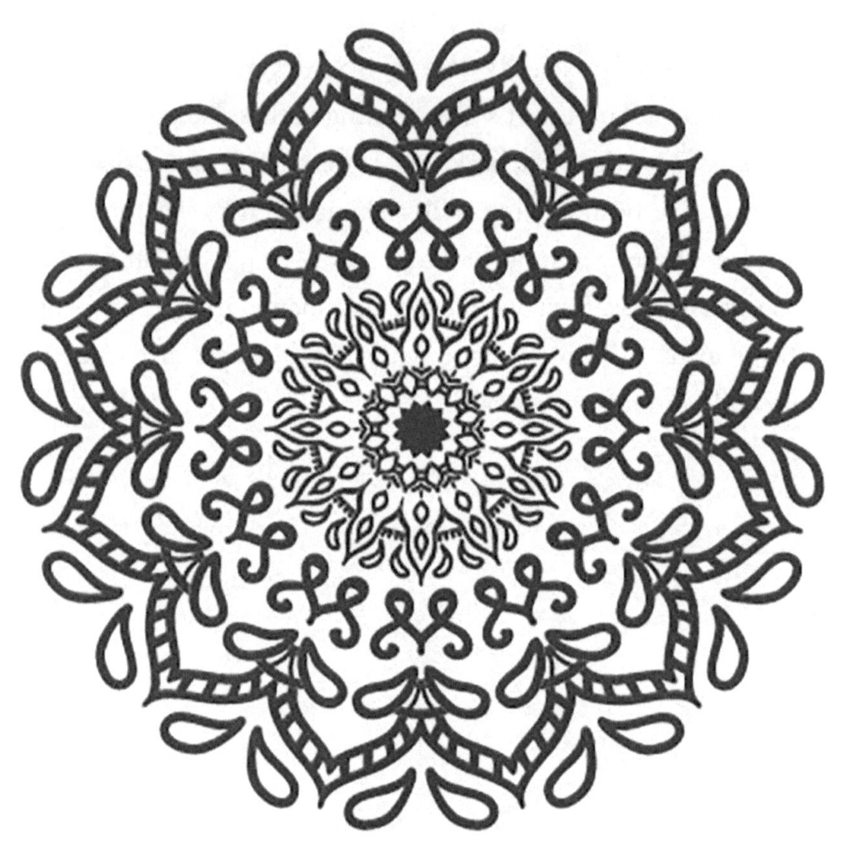

Morning in My Life

By Writer Jennifer Bartholomew from Illinois, USA

> *"When you have lost hope, you have lost everything. And when you think all is lost, when all is dire and bleak, there is always hope".*
> ~Pittacus Lore

I woke up at 3am to myself crying. In my dream I was sitting next to the ocean, toes in the sand and waves crashing. I was enjoying the sunlight beaming on my skin, breathing deep the salty air. Suddenly the clouds split open and the light faded as a thunderstorm broke. Lightning was blasting my body, multiple areas at once. I began to spasm and shake like I was having a seizure, pain crippling my joints and electricity burrowing into my bones. Flames licked at my frame, burning my muscles and my skin. All I could do was collapse and watch in horror as I succumbed to my injuries. I heard myself crying in real life, but in my dream, it seemed to be coming from the seagulls that bombed me, picking off one body part at a time. Slowly my conscience mind became aware, and I opened my eyes, still feeling the burning, electric pain coursing through me.

Every movement I attempted amplified the agony, I felt like I was stuck in between worlds, the dream world misting over reality like a haze. My brain yelled at me to move, sit up, roll over!!! Do something to break this stream of unconsciousness that was holding me under. All I could do was cry. I felt the hot tears rolling down my face and neck, I could taste the salty drops running over my lips. Finally, I knew what was happening, it happened too many times to count. During sleep, pain levels began soaring as they always do, penetrating my subconscious, rendering me an invalid as I desperately tried to free myself from the nightmare, I actually live every day.

Eyes open and fully aware, my body is locked. I try to lift an arm or roll myself over to my back but no matter how many times I tell my body to listen, my demands go unheard, communication is broken between mind and body. So, I stay still. I close my eyes to go back to the darkness, quenching the fears that maybe this time is "THE" time, the last time my body will move on its own.

Taking inventory and being used to this type of event, I slow my breathing. Deep, long breaths in through my nose, slowly exhaled through my mouth. I have to slow my heart rate; I can feel my hypertension is rampant and in order to calm down I have to regain control. Desperately praying for the pain to cease, I keep doing breath work while I search for any part of me that can move....I wiggle my toes.

Opening my eyes again I slowly, gingerly slide my arms out to the wall and press my sweaty palms on the cool drywall, rocking back and forth until I have enough momentum to push my body on its back. Arms at my sides, I take an inventory of everything that is hurting as pain pulses through my entire body like my blood itself. No longer audibly crying, I still notice tears dripping off my cheekbones.

I decide to stay in this position, just rolling over has exhausted me and my pulse is high. I place my two fingers on the opposite wrist and count...heart rate 168 upon waking. For most this would be alarming, for me it's tolerable. Just resting my heart rate usually sits at 115-120. Just another one of the hundreds of symptoms that come along with my illnesses. I flush my system with water, staring out into my room like it's a travel destination, doing all I can do to not fall victim to yet another day of the symptoms and the gut-wrenching pain that is my life.

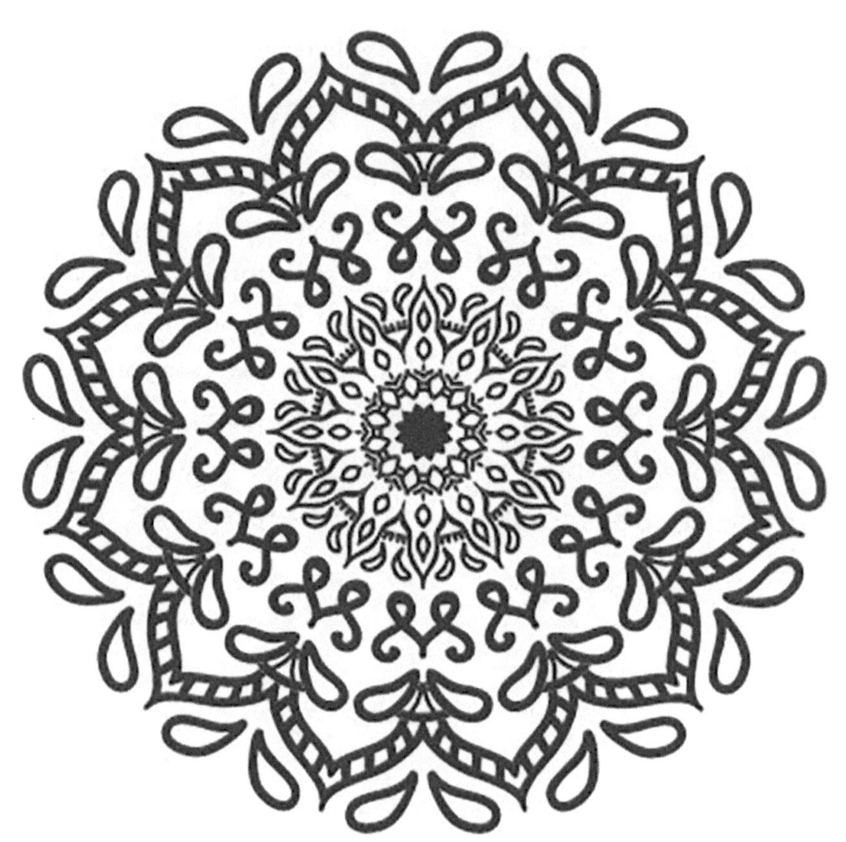

Anguish Day-To-Day

By Writer
Deborah Denise Lafeber Macias from Texas, USA

"Strength and growth come only through continuous effort and struggle."
~Napoleon Hill

I have come a long way in learning, the hard way, of course, that there's a reason for everything, good or bad, that happens to me. I have had numerous different, horrible sufferings and struggles in my life, literally for as long as I can remember, starting when I was only five years old. But I have continuously put in persistent efforts to strive and thrive for a better life. I had always doubted the phrase "what doesn't kill you makes you stronger" crap that I was always told, and I hated hearing it, but I guess it's true in a way. Because I have finally realized that I have grown in knowledge and wisdom from living in this difficult world, as well as acquired a powerful strength as a result of all

I've endured over the years. I now know that I am a very strong woman and a survivor multiple times over and over.

I'm guessing that since I have not died, either by my attempts or from my ill health, that it just means that God isn't done with me for whatever reason. Having so much wrong with me physically, mentally, emotionally, and spiritually has led me to be so very hungry and desperate for a more deeply intimate relationship with our Lord God, because I desperately desire to feel His pure joy and the Holy Spirit's warmth, enjoy the comfort of Jesus Christ holding me in His arms when I am in His presence. Only God knows everything that I am literally suffering and struggling with. Although these illnesses and chronic fatigue is invisible to other people, they are visible to God. People just don't understand when I say I just don't feel good and I am just too tired for this or that.

I have moved away from my hometown from all those doctors and specialists that had diagnosed me and was helping me little by little to feel well and somewhat normal, whatever that really is. So many doctors and specialists don't really want to listen to me, and I have had to change from some bad ones that have told me to shut up. One of them was the reason I almost died when my whole body became very septic - twice in two different months with an emergency surgery in between.

I have been to doctors or specialists and given a list to them and they were like, wait let's just deal with one or two things for right now. I just don't feel listened to, then they just want to prescribe more medications on top of the many I already have to take, and I hate all the awful side effects. I've been told that they can't give me anything for my fibromyalgia or anything else until I see psych! That just gets me upset. It makes me feel like they believe that all my pain is just in my head, that it's psychological. I was told that this or that test was a false positive, so they referred me to psych because they think that would help this ailment, or that I just need to be put on antidepressants again since it's all in my medical history.

There is no cure for this awful chronic fatigue syndrome, but I have found that keeping to a routine sleep cycle by going to bed at night and waking in the morning around the same time every day and even on weekends, helps. Of course, I'm not always following that routine because many different things happen each day, and I am more of a night owl than a morning early bird person. I also suffer with insomnia kind of bad sometimes.

I must force myself to not over work myself and not do anything overly strenuous, well to me these days everything seems too hard and strenuous. But I had to learn how my body has changed with everything that's wrong with it, and if I push myself too much or too hard for too long, then I will just crash. Then I will have no other option, but to lay down and rest. Unfortunately, any amount of rest doesn't help me, and if I over did any kind of work, then most likely I won't make it out of bed the next day or even longer.

I have to listen to my body and give it what it needs to feel better. My prayers to God, my faith, believing and trusting that He is my healer, my physician, and of course my everything. I know I am a survivor because of God, who strengthens me every split second of each minute of the long days, and I will conquer this terrible chronic fatigue syndrome by changing my lifestyle for the better. I will work on eating more natural organic foods, the way God intended for us to eat. All the processed foods that are manmade, unhealthy crap that I fed my body, has over time made me sick.

I believe from what I've researched about this hard invisible disease, that it has been linked to candida, anemia, hormonal imbalance, low thyroid, viral infections, allergies, nutritional deficiencies, parasites, and whatever toxicities from food and chemical pollutants, and too much stress, just to name a few. In conclusion, I just must change my eating habits, keep to a better sleep routine, go out and get my daily walk or light exercise, and some natural sun to help my vitamin D deficiency, and of course just keep praying.

Author Bios

Writer Bio – Kari Ainslie from Espanola, Ontario

Kari graduated from Nipissing University with an Honors English degree and Bachelor of Education. After a couple years working in a daycare, she pursued more education by obtaining an Early Childhood Education diploma. In September 2014, she was hired at a Christian school to teach Kindergarten. However, it was that winter (February 2015) that she became ill. Kari never knew that illness would last to this current day. She is currently diagnosed with chronic fatigue syndrome as well as irritable bowel syndrome. These diagnoses have changed her life path. One thing that has been important and beneficial for Kari is to connect with other people who are struggling with chronic illness, to offer support, compassion, and talk to someone else who "gets it." She hopes to do just that by sharing her stories.

Writer Bio ~

Deborah Denise Lafeber Macias from Texas, USA

Deborah Denise Lafeber- Macias is 47 years of age. She currently lives in San Antonio, Texas and she was born and raised in Amarillo, Texas. She's an entrepreneur as a Paparazzi $5.00 Jewelry & Accessories Consultant and she even has her own website, it's www.paparazziaccessories.com/227644. A little story behind her maiden name Lafeber is it was originally spelled as Lefebere and she remembers that's what her Dad had told her many years ago, but now that her Dad passed away her Mom had told her that her Dad's original last name was really Lafebere. But her Dad said to her Mom that he didn't like it, so he just changed it, on his own without doing it the legal way. His Dad was upset with him because of it for years! She knows he just changed the first "e" to an "a" and then left off the last "e" but she doesn't know how he got away with it though, but she always thought of her Dad as a rebel. Deborah is a single Mom blessed with three precious children that God has lent to her. Deborah was born into a catholic religion family, but she had felt that she wasn't being spiritually fed and in her early 30's she started her own journey to find God through Christianity. She found many Christian teachings, preaching's, and praying on television that she enjoyed watching and hearing Pastors preach & teach the Holy Bible to where she could understand everything way better and to where she can apply it all to her own life, and how to live it how God planned. She searched for a good spiritual feeding Christian Faith Church. Deborah has a daughter named Kierastyn Denise Lafeber Razura and she's 26 years of age and married with a successful career as a massage therapist and is attending college classes to become a physical therapist. Deborah also has a son named Zeric Jaden Lafeber and he is 18 years of age and has just graduated high school a year and a half ahead of schedule. Her youngest sons is named Xavier Jett Macias and he is starting 9th grade in a new high school and he is finally getting to be in JROTC which stands for Junior Reserve Officers Training Corps and he has been wanting to join the class since he saw them outside at his sister's high school years ago. When Xavier was just 2 1/2 years old he had told his Momma something so precious and mind boggling while at the DMV he pointed up at the Marine's pamphlets where it showed men in sharp looking uniforms and amongst all the Military services he chose that specific one and said "Momma that's what I gonna be when I groweded bigger!" She is just so very proud of all her adorable, precious, loving children that God has trusted her with despite all she was suffering and she feels her babies really saved her life literally and she is so very grateful to God for loving her and trusting her so much that He has lent His precious children to her to teach, guide, nurture, love and care for them with His unconditional love. Her parent's names are John Domingo Lafeber and Juanita Delia Montoya Lafeber. Her Dad sadly passed away from congestive heart failure, type two diabetes this year on January 31st, 2019 he was 72, Deborah's Moms age is 71 now and it's been so heartbreaking for her. Deborah worked long, tough hours at a maximum-security men's prison in Amarillo, Tx., so she can provide for her three children after an abrupt divorce. Deborah has hopes and dreams of someday soon to travel the world.

Author Susan Parker Rosen from Maryland, USA

Start with a Blank Piece of Paper!

Susan Parker Rosen is a Self-Published Author that did not start writing her first novella until age 60. In a dream, one of her Aunts hugged her and told her to "start with a blank piece of paper," the next day she did just that.

Her latest fiction novella, "Cold Case in Cape May," She wanted to write about that amazing town since she grew up there as a child going there each summer to visit family. It's written about a quirky gal Izzy, who visits an old childhood friend in that town, while leaving her family at home, and they both end up becoming a sleuth to solve a mystery that is a couple decades old. There are no real graphic details, it's filled with humor as well as heart breaking pages. Cape May is a beautiful setting and part of the book is set in scenic Long Neck De, where the author resided up until approximately 5 years ago. Even Izzy's Pug gets involved in this Cozy Mystery!

Susan Parker Rosen herself struggles with fibromyalgia, a disorder of the central nervous system. This is what she had to say about this book, "The Many Faces of Fibro – The Special Love Edition," I've struggled with fibro since being involved in a major car accident in 1991, after being thrown from a vehicle. Luckily my life was spared, as I landed on a small plot of grass that was surrounded by concrete and highway. Lucky isn't even the word for it, so if I need to live a life of pain, I look at it as part of my life that I'm fortunate to have. I'm here and I'm breathing! But that in no way will ever stop me from enjoying life – the best that I can. This books' goal as explained in the introduction. Is to give those with fibro support with travel, if you are fearful of what others may think of you when you make mistakes while vacationing, you will see you are not the only one. Maybe you didn't have any "flip-flop" trips that go awry, just seeing that other people are just like us and have struggles with being away from all the comforts of home with a challenging disorder.

Although fibromyalgia is usually not diagnosed until the signature flare pain starts, Susan's own opinion is that she has had this disorder for as long as she can remember. "Other things were always going on that made me feel different from other people I knew. In my teens and 20s I was always extremely tired. Slept often and never felt as if I had a refreshed sleep. I would drag myself along through the day, couple all that with a desire to succeed in business. I was always achieving more and enjoying life less. My home life suffered, caused two divorces and I never really had 'real fulfillment' people normally receive from relationships, this continued until I was able to recognize that this is part of the disorder and that I could make positive changes in my life."

Today, with her writing Susan feels a strong desire to continue healing, not only herself but others with the stories within these pages. "I may always have this disorder, or hopefully they will find a cure, but at age 68 I'm not going to give up! I can work from the comfort of my bedroom, even from bedside if need be. Typing is accomplished on my small notebook and I use a website to find freelance jobs and I'm able to earn extra income and feel as if I'm contributing to society."

Her passion for writing drives her to continue putting together a continuing series on fibro as well as other invisible disorders/disease's, until awareness is widespread. Not just for the people that are in her life, but people in the lives of all strugglers' around the world.

Susan resides on the Eastern Shore of Maryland in a small historic town known as Pocomoke City Md. The home that she shares with her husband Tim Latham was built before the turn of the century. When you come to our town it is as if taking a step back in time. I came here to semi-retire and to enjoy writing in a friendly, laid- back town filled with history and nature. It's perfect!

Reach out to her and if you have an interest in writing, you will find that she is always happy to help. If you struggle with one of these disorders, she believes you can find freedom from feeling trapped by chronic illness simply by "starting with a blank piece of paper!"

You can read more about the author Susan Parker Rosen,

Also, stop by and join our Facebook group, "101fibro – The many Faces of Fibro" our group is comprised of others that struggle, and you can join feeling comfortable that no one will judge you and you will feel a comfort within a supportive group that know just what you are going through. Our upcoming books are normally posted there.

If you are curious about what we are doing and how easy it is to tell your story and become published email me! I'll give you the information you need to get started. Every story is important and costs you nothing to be a part of the program.

Other groups are being developed for other invisible diseases/disorders. Our books that are open for submission will be listed in the rear of this book as well as the corresponding FB group. Join those groups for all updated details including the deadline for submissions.

Reach out to Susan Parker Rosen by emailing her anytime. Let us know your thoughts on our books and if we can help support you in your struggle with fibro or other invisible diseases/disorders. We will tell you about our exciting incentive program!

Author Bio ~ Robin Dix from Maine, USA

Robin Dix has suffered with CFS for many years along with multiple other chronic illnesses. She works hard at keeping a positive mindset, as she believes that gives her hope and the ability to cope better.

She is married with three grown children and one spoiled cat. She enjoys computer games, reading, good coffee, and hanging out with family and friends.

She began her writing career over three years ago. She was looking for a way to generate some income from home, as she was mostly bed bound. She writes a weekly column and has authored or co-authored 3 books so far. She began editing and proofreading a year ago. As an avid reader she is quick to pick up spelling and grammatical errors.

She considers it a huge blessing that God has gifted her in this.

Writer Bio ~ Candace Kay from Delaware, USA

Candace Kay was born in south eastern Pennsylvania in 1968, to a blue-collar family. Suffering from various conditions as a child, illnesses progressed, all would come to light in her 40's, as things would be properly diagnosed. Married and divorced two times, Ms. Kay resides in a seaside town in Lower Slower Delaware with her faithful companions, Toby and Abby her beloved dogs.

Her hobbies include reading, writing, crocheting, knitting, cooking, offering education and support to others that have chronic illnesses, and spending as much time as she can with her grandchildren. She connected with various groups on the internet, and finally decided to write about her journey with CFS and other diseases.

She is finally fulfilling her dream of writing and helping people understand various autoimmune and neurologic diseases.

Writer Bio ~
Asha Ryan from Ramsbottom, Lancashire, UK

Hello. My name is Asha Ryan. I am 42 years old and live in a pretty little town in the North of England, called Ramsbottom. I moved here, from the city of Manchester with my fabulous and amazing husband of 8 years and our beautiful daughter who's 6.

Whilst in Manchester I forged a successful career in the corporate world and had my own business as a Complementary Therapist. I was sociable too and my husband and I enjoyed exploring new places to eat and drink in the city with friends new and old. We'd got married and become parents too.

Sadly, part way through these wonderful experiences I got CFS after a bout of Glandular Fever and had to give up my job.

Life was a real struggle when I first became ill on a physical, mental, emotional and spiritual level. I was off sick from work. My fiancé was away working, I was trying to plan our wedding and I was battling Depression.

It was about this time that I found God, or should I say he found me. He found me through a prophesizing Christian friend who shared my passion for Reiki and holistic therapies.

Although the CFS still impacts basic aspects of my life significantly, 50% of the time I can function with mild symptoms in a fairly normal capacity and I am sure I have God to thank for that healing.

I no longer feel guided to work as a complementary therapist, instead I am focusing on looking after myself and being the best mum I can to our daughter, but it was through my work as a holistic therapist that I came to feel my life purpose was in helping others.

I am not sure what the next part of my journey looks like, so I guess I'll continue to pray and see what happens. What I do know is it will be worth it.

Author Bio – Donna Short RN from Michigan, USA

Donna lives in Michigan with her wonderful husband of 7 years, and their 2 spoiled dogs. She also has 2 amazing adult children Raven her son and Jadyn her daughter, they are such a blessing! As of February 2014, she became physically unable to work as a home health care registered nurse any longer. She has kept her nursing license active and she keeps her continuing education requirements up to date, including her CPR basic life support. She plans to keep her licenses active because she has a hope for a cure one day. She is currently on disability as of 2016, and she is learning everyday how to manage her fibromyalgia so that she can live her best life. Fibromyalgia is a part of, but she is not fibromyalgia, she is a fighter and will fight for others and herself to remove the stigma that fibromyalgia brings with it. She will continue to be a voice of advocacy, education and teaching, along with the voice of how to once again love yourself despite fibromyalgia.

Donna is also an advocate and volunteer yearly for the Annual Alzheimer's Walk here in Flint, Michigan https://www.alz.org/gmc for her father who passed from the disease. She is currently working closely with the Fibromyalgia Association of Michigan

https://www.facebook.com/MiFibromyalgia/

On starting a Fibromyalgia Support Group in her area, she stated "we don't have many resources in my area, and it would be a great assess." Donna attends many free seminars at

https://medicine.umich.edu/dept/cpfrc/resources

Online to learn all she can about fibromyalgia, so she is well educated and can become an excellent advocate and educator to the public and for people suffering with this disease. She aspires to become a public speaker for the chronically ill. Donna has her own blog called "Healing with Donna Short RN." https://donnashortrn.com Donna helps the chronically ill heal with food. She is on her own healing journey. Donna states that "If it wasn't for God's mercy and provision, she would not be able to do all she does! She does the best she can every day, she listens to her body and cares for it with love and forgiveness, she also visualizes her highest self, then starts showing up as that person."

Author Bio ~ Jeanne Pallos from California, USA

Jeanne Pallos is a published author with several stories in the Chicken Soup for the Soul series. She has struggled with CFS all her adult life yet chooses to not let it define her. She has been blessed with a very loving, supportive husband who has never doubted her illness. She lives in Laguna Niguel, CA with her husband of 46 years. They have two grown children and two grandchildren.

Writer Bio ~
Jennifer Bartholomew from Illinois, USA

Born in Illinois, Jennifer Bartholomew spent her younger years in Texas, followed by a move back to Illinois where she currently lives. At ten years old she discovered her love for writing. From short stories to poems, she wrote what she felt, lived, and dreamed.

A mother of five beautiful children and grandma to one, her life consisted of being the best mom she could be, always desiring to one day reach others with her words.

When ME/CFS and other illnesses changed the way she lived life, writing became the tool to cope with the difference between healthy and chronic living. She aspires to one day helping others who live and battle with chronic pain and illness, hoping that what she has experienced can be beneficial for those who desire to live abundantly, despite their challenges.

Writer Bio – Gargi Sanyal from India

Gargi, in my words is ~
"A warrior in the garden and not just a gardener in the war".
~Gargi Sanyal

She believes that learning never ends, so goes on learning, and preparing herself always and growing up with the right values and right knowledge. She runs after her passions like a butterfly while never allows the child within herself to die. She dreams to live life to her fullest and enjoys every moment of it. Miraculously behind every negative she finds out a positive and motivates herself as well as others. I have never seen her falling and not getting up again, being broken. She has an immense faith in God and an unshakable belief that the world is driven by and only by love, truth, honesty, humanity and righteousness.

She includes these as the only basic points of living, in the teachings to her two sweetie-naughty daughters – Indrakshi and Yuvakshi. She believes children should be raised with these values instead of the way they are raised nowadays and also we the adults, the more we grow, we kill the child within us and become complex minded and inhumane, instead of staying innocent, humane, loving and true, ultimately forgetting the purpose of one's life.

She was a teacher throughout her career of 14 years after which she had to quit her job owing to family issues initially and finally on diagnosis of her disability of Fibromyalgia. She is a passionate lady, in one sentence – 'Jack of all trades.' She loves to sing, to dance, to play piano, to sketch her thoughts, to write quotes, stories and poems, to recite and act in plays, to make handicrafts, to cook exiting dishes in funny ways. She is also very compassionate and loving, so by nature motivates others and fights for the truth, humanity and justice by actively participating as an activist as per her feasibility.

As her husband, I have no shame today to admit that I too took time to recognize her properly but, the greatest quality which I found in her is that - she doesn't believe in punishments given by human, rather she believes in making every negative turn into a positive. She believes in spreading love, self-realization and awareness. She believes God is always present within them who never gives up trying to live. I don't fear today to admit she had been tortured a lot by many including me, before she was diagnosed with fibromyalgia owing to our unawareness and some ill practices of society, but she didn't give up. In India, Invisible diseases like fibromyalgia and chronic fatigue syndrome are still mostly unknown and there are lot of wrong beliefs and malpractices superimposed even in this 21st century. People here, need to be awarded through right education and the society needs to be changed. She believes in 'Life of Significance than Life of Success' and aspires to work for the people, for the society, on all levels with her strong self-belief that-

'Andhokar sarani dhore sesh hobe e path chola, Aasbe jeno sei Sokal Jiboneri galpo bola...'

~ (verses of a Bengali song meaning- 'Walking through this dark road will end someday, be sure – the dawn will come to narrate the story of life one day'...).

Last but not the least, from the eyes of an human and not from that of her husband, I can say, the way she has been able to change me from my darker side to my brighter one, it is not very far when she will be able to succeed to see her dreams with her open eyes and, we all together hand in hand, one day will be able to make a new horizon of better mankind.
~Tonmoy

"I wholeheartedly express my gratitude to Invisible Publications for giving me an opportunity to make a part of my dream come true. I also feel myself to be blessed to be part of the team." **~Gargi**

Writer Bio – Charmaine from Australia

Charmaine is from Australia, recently turned 61. She is a born-again Christian (very important in her life) She is happily divorced and has a daughter and a son who both have two gorgeous boys each. Her daughter is only 10 minutes away from her, and her son is a 12-hour drive away. Charmaine likes to drive once a year to where her son and his family live, but her fatigue is worse and, unfortunately, that is not happening this year.

As she has written, she does pick up her grandsons after school, and she feels so blessed to be able to be involved in their lives. Fibromyalgia and ME/CFS has a lot of symptoms. One of them is chronic pain. For Charmaine's pain management she scrapbooks, and enjoys card making and quilting. It takes her mind off whatever is going on, and especially the pain.

Author Bio - Abby Guss from Ohio, USA

Abby Guss is a classically trained singer, actor, published model, author and voice over artist who has been on stage since she was small. She has performed all over the United States in front of thousands of people, most notably at the Ryman Auditorium. She is a staunch supporter of philanthropy, women's rights and access to affordable and proper healthcare. While she suffers with a chronic autoimmune illness, she still tries to focus on positivity and living life with love and gratitude.

Outside of anything in the arts, her hobbies include cooking, hiking, and traveling. You can find her at her blog and podcast, Not a Face for Radio.